STO

3.4.80

SELF HEALTH

SELF HEALTH

The Lifelong Fitness Book

Nathaniel Lande

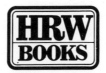

Holt, Rinehart and Winston
New York

For Robert Greenblatt M.D.—
friend and father,
physician and philosopher—
with thanks

ACKNOWLEDGMENTS

The author wishes to thank his editor, Carolyn Trager, and his publisher, David Mendelsohn; and to express warm and special appreciation to George Maldonaldo, Marylou Vaughn, and Douglas Colligan, whose research, organization, and direction helped create this book. Lastly, the author wishes to acknowledge the work of Dr. Kaare Norum, whose scientific inquiry has been a major contribution to the field of health and nutrition.

Library of Congress Cataloging in Publication Data

Lande, Nathaniel.
    Self-Health: The Lifelong Fitness Book

    1. Physical fitness.   2. Exercise.   3. Nutrition.
I.   Title.
RA781.L348   613.7   79–14671
ISBN 0–03–048316–6

Printed in the United States of America
10 9 8 7 6 5 4 3 2 1

CONTENTS

1

GUIDELINES TO A HEALTHY FUTURE

Too many of us seem to think we have little control over the state of our health. We tend to blame many of our health problems on things like the toxins in our environment, the silent viruses and microbes that invade our bodies, even the additives in our food. We also tend to think the process of getting and staying healthy is simply a matter of seeing the doctor when we're sick and getting that magic pill or drug to cure us.

In fact, good health has little to do with doctors and even less to do with pills or drugs. Good health is largely a matter of habit. Dr. John H. Knowles of the Rockefeller Foundation stated that: "Your health is your own doing. It depends overwhelmingly on what you do today. And what you did yesterday. And what you do tomorrow. Nothing drastic. Just your everyday personal habits. Simple basic things like a sensible diet, exercise, not too much drinking, enough rest, no smoking.

"You don't believe it? Then take a look at the percentages. Only about *10 percent* of human health can be affected by the medical system—and that goes for doctors, medications, hospitals, surgery—the works. The other 90 percent is determined by things over which doctors have little or no control—and that really means your personal habits."

It's as simple as that.

Yet few of us ever really take the time to sit down and think about developing those habits that can give us that 90 percent control over our health. Why? Part of the answer lies in human nature. Good health is important to all of us, but like most good things in life, we never really notice it until it's gone, until we get sick. Then, when we've recovered from our ailment, we make all kinds of promises to ourselves and our loved ones: to quit smoking, drink less, eat less, skip desserts, take up jogging, eat nothing but celery, reform totally—all in about two weeks. Sound familiar?

What usually happens is that by the third week we find ourselves smoking again, partly because we also never really stopped drinking, and we always smoked when we drank. The vow to skip all desserts dissolved at the first sight of a soft, rich chocolate mousse; the all-celery diet turned out to be less exciting than it sounded; and even with a nifty running suit and a new pair of sky blue nylon running shoes, jogging was hard work. Our legs hurt too much, so we stopped. We weren't sick any more, so why worry?

Even if you conquer this problem, there is the more complex one of getting decent, reliable information on what a person can do to get in the habit of good health. The shelves of bookstores are filled with diet books that guarantee you can lose ten pounds in one week and still eat anything you want, or that promise to take inches off your waistline in a few days. But there's more to good health than just losing pounds. If being skinny were the only criterion, famine victims should be the healthiest people on the planet.

You also can read piles of books on whatever the latest exercise fad is. The problem with these is that while they may tell you how to get stronger, run faster, tone up a flabby body, few give sound advice on what to put into that body. Knowing how to push your body to finish a marathon without getting a heart attack is not all that valuable on a day-to-day basis. Neither is being able to lose thirty pounds on a diet of, say, nothing but cheesecake and seltzer water. The problem with most fads, in exercises or diet, is that even if they do what they claim, they do not give most of us what we really want, a guide to long and healthy life. With the hundreds of books written on getting and staying healthy, none offers a truly comprehensive life plan of good health habits that will work for you as well when you are thirty-five as when you are seventy-five. Only *Self-Health* does.

What is self-health? It is a simple, easy-to-understand and easy-to-follow program of eating and fitness that uses the very latest discoveries in nutrition and exercise. It's a sane and simple way of getting that 90 percent control over your health and well-being. Self-health uses no gadgets, no gimmicks, no special foods, and no resources other than common sense and good science. The program is easy to master and highly adaptable. It can be customized to suit your life style with little problem.

By following the self-health way of living you will:

- reduce certain risk factors that tend to age and wear down the human body
- extend your healthy life span by as much as fifteen years
- increase your natural energy, vitality, and endurance

9

- enjoy all the benefits of a trim, youthful, and nutritionally sound body.

And you can achieve all this in just twelve weeks.

Very simply, the self-health program is made up of two parts. The first is a carefully designed nutrition plan which you can shape and customize to your particular needs. The second is an exercise plan designed to bring you up to and keep you at your peak of physical fitness. Both parts are designed to help you survive and thrive in today's environment. All you need to take advantage of the program are the willingness to try and a little knowledge about yourself.

GET TO KNOW YOUR BODY

Your body is unique. It is a product of a dizzying variety of influences: your personal genetic makeup, your biochemistry, your life style, your diet, your exercise habits (or lack of them), your environment. Before you can begin to plan an intelligent self-health program for yourself, you have to know a little bit about all these influences that help make you what you are.

Start with your genetic inheritance. Contained in everyone is DNA, a genetic blueprint inherited from both parents. DNA is a protein substance that relays certain inherited physical "information" to genes which in turn carry it along from one generation to the next. This genetic code contains everything from the color of your hair and eyes to your body's disposition to certain strengths and weaknesses. If, for example, your father had a history of heart disease, there's a good possibility you could be predisposed to it as well. In instances like this, knowing your family's and your parents' medical history can alert you to possible trouble spots in your system and help you decide what special protective measures to take to live a healthy life. In this case keeping careful watch over your blood pressure and moderating the stresses in your life will help balance out the inborn tendency to heart disease. Some scientists feel it is even possible to change some of these genetic tendencies by the way we manage our health. Over and over again, studies have shown that a healthy diet and a healthy environment produce healthier parents. They in turn have healthier children. For this reason, taking the time to make some of these changes for the better would not only benefit you now, but could also be a legacy of health you could pass on to future generations.

Another very basic part of your whole body health is what you put into it—your diet. The more experts study diet, the more they learn about the breadth and depth of its effect on your health. To give an extreme example, there is a tribe called the Hunzas in Northern Tibet who are remarkable for their longevity and vitality. They have active sex lives well into their nineties and many live to be over a hundred. They're a remarkably fit people rarely afflicted by the diseases and ailments that plague so-called more advanced societies. Doctors who studied them found one main reason for their amazing stamina. It was their diet. The Hunzas eat little meat, eat nothing that has been refined or processed, and get most of their nutrients from raw vegetables, fruits, yogurt, sprouted beans, and whole grain flour. As you will see in Chapter Three some of their diet has been incorporated into the self-health program.

Until very recently anyone who dared to make such a connection between the Hunzas' long and healthy lives and their diet would have been branded as some sort of health-food nut. But this attitude has changed. Today there are a growing number of nutrition specialists, some of whom work for the U.S. Department of Agriculture, who are saying that hundreds of thousands of lives could be saved each year simply by improving our diets. Among the improvements they say could be made by dietary changes are:

- Reduction of the cancer rate by 20 to 40 percent
- Heart disease reduced by 25 to 50 percent
- Dental problems reduced by 50 percent
- Significantly fewer birth defects
- Cure rate for schizophrenia increased by as much as 500 percent
- Far fewer problems with arthritis, allergies, digestive problems, diabetes, and even alcoholism
- Increased longevity and vitality for all.

These predictions, all founded on sound scientific research, should give you an idea of just how powerfully nutrition can affect your life. Unfortunately, nutrition is one of the most overlooked and least understood factors in our health lives. We are apt to know more about, and pay more attention to, our cars than our bodies. Remember, you can always get a new car if the one you own breaks down. You don't have the luxury of that choice with your body.

HOW TO GAUGE YOUR OWN SELF-HEALTH

Unfortunately, we ourselves are the cause of much of what erodes the quality of our health. Fortunately, some of the damage is within our control and is reversible. You probably already know what those wear-and-tear habits are, and have at least a vague notion of what they can do to you. It's hard to remain ignorant of at least some of the effects of smoking, of being overweight, of being a heavy drinker, of living or working in high-stress situations. What you tend *not* to think about is the cumulative effect of all these factors on your health and, ultimately, your life. The first step towards self-health is to sit yourself down and make a list of risk factors in your life—habits and situations that are basically antihealth. You can't plan any realistic improvements in health unless you can first get some general idea of the kind of shape you're in right now.

RISK FACTORS

Ideally, your first step in the direction of self-health is to eliminate or reduce the following risk factors from your life:

- Smoking
- Overeating
- Heavy drinking
- Stress

At this point it might be helpful to review just *why* all these qualify as risk factors.

Smoking

According to current statistics there are 50 million smokers in the United States, roughly 30 percent of the men and 29 percent of all the women in this country. Why do they smoke? Well, the reasons vary but the ones most commonly given are:

- "It's just a habit."
- "I'm addicted."
- "It gives me a little boost of energy."
- "It helps me relax and enjoy a meal."

- "I've just got to have something in my hands all the time."

In spite of these "benefits" many smokers today are worried. And for good reason. They have to deal not only with the rising concern about their health from their families, the increasingly more open and widespread hostility from nonsmokers, and growing restrictions on when and where they can smoke, but with an impressively grim catalogue of the hazards as well.

For one thing, a smoker stands an increased risk of contracting emphysema, a serious lung disorder which has no cure. What happens with this disease is that individual lung cells lose their elasticity and cannot contract properly to let out air after each breath. Breathing becomes increasingly difficult and the disease places a tremendous strain on the heart.

As anyone who has seen a lung-association ad knows, smoking also increases the odds of getting lung cancer, a major killer of men and the third most prevalent type of cancer among women. Studies have shown that compared to nonsmokers, moderate smokers are eight times as likely to get this cancer and heavy smokers are twenty times as susceptible.

Smoking has also been found to be a contributing factor in heart disease. Exactly how it affects the heart is still not clear, but two important factors appear to be nicotine and carbon monoxide, both plentiful in cigarette smoke. Nicotine is known to raise blood pressure and increase the heart's demand for oxygen. Carbon monoxide aggravates these effects by decreasing the blood's ability to furnish that needed oxygen.

It is also known that smoke damages the cilia, the delicate hairlike projections that line the bronchial tubes.

With these damaged or destroyed, the lungs lose an early line of defense against infections.

Studies have also shown that smokers tend to have about a 20 percent higher incidence of stroke than non-smokers, a risk that increases if a smoker also has high blood pressure or high cholesterol. Lastly, smoking has other more subtle effects as well. It interferes with your body's ability to use vitamin C and for some reason also interferes with the beneficial effects of pain-killing and anxiety-reducing drugs.

Now the obvious alternative to exposing yourself to these health hazards is not to start smoking or to quit if you already are. Unfortunately, that is not always so easy. If you are a smoker, you have only two choices. The ideal one of course is to give up smoking and eliminate this risk factor from your life completely. If you can't or won't quit, you have to accept the risks and the health deficits that come with it.

Overeating

Overeating and its natural consequence, being overweight, is a slightly more insidious problem you may have had to handle at one time or another. It's not really something you set out to do to yourself deliberately, like taking up smoking. Quite often it just seems to happen. One of the most common ways it sneaks up on us is as part of the aging process. Usually as people get older their lives become more sedentary, less physically demanding, and their need for calories drops because they are generating less energy. Since this does not happen all of a sudden, people sometimes are unaware of it and continue the same eating habits they had when they were younger and much more active. Or they even may have shifted their eating habits in the wrong direction: having between meal snacks, drinking an extra 150 or 200 calories in the form of a beer or mixed drink as they watch television. Before they know it their clothes don't fit quite so well, and they don't feel so light.

But age is only part of the cause. Living in an affluent society takes its toll on our waistline and ultimately our health. According to Dr. Theodore VanItallie, head of a special weight-control program funded by the National Institute of Health at St. Luke's Hospital in New York City, "Obesity is a predicament of people in affluent societies. To some extent it represents a loss of control, a victimization of the individual by his environment. . . ."

And victims we are. Being overweight is an especially tough health problem. It affects the whole person. People who are overweight or obese are often self-conscious about their weight. They have a bad self-image and in many cases may be openly discriminated against because they are fat. Obesity often draws people into a vicious circle. They are miserable because they eat too much and they eat too much because they are miserable.

Being overweight is a real health hazard as well. For one thing it is much tougher for overweight people to motivate themselves to exercise than it is for someone who is out of shape but close to an ideal weight. And staying overweight raises the possibility of other, deadly health problems. Someone who is 25 percent over his or her ideal body weight, researchers have found, is two and a half times more likely to have a heart attack than someone at normal weight.

There are several reasons for this. One is the simple physical fact that obesity puts an extra circulatory load on your heart. Blood volume increases with weight and all of a sudden your heart has to pump out more blood to fat that wasn't there before.

Because of your fatty diet you might also be taking the risk of raising your cholesterol level to dangerous highs. A diet of high-fat, cholesterol-rich foods can bring about atherosclerosis, or hardening of the arteries, an especially volatile condition if you have a family history of heart attack or stroke. If your doctor has checked your cholesterol level and it's over 180, now is the time to start thinking about changing your life and your diet.

Another contributing factor to heart problems is high blood pressure. This is a silent risk factor that often has no symptoms and only makes itself known with a heart attack. Over a period of time it enlarges and weakens the heart and helps speed up the process of hardening of the arteries in which the blood vessels' inner walls narrow and fill with fatty deposits.

The best and simplest way to find out your blood pressure is to have a doctor take it or get the inflatable cuff and reading unit and take it yourself. Blood pressure can vary to some extent from day to day. The acceptable average pressure is usually considered to be 140/90 (for 140 systolic pressure over 90 diastolic). A pressure lower than that is even better for decreasing the risk of a stroke or heart attack. The lowest risk comes with 120/80 or less.

Another complication that can come with obesity is diabetes, too high a level of blood sugar. Those particularly susceptible to it are the offspring of diabetics. But although some people have an inherited susceptibility to the disease, many cases almost certainly are brought on by a sugar-heavy diet. In our country where the sugar consumption per person averages ninety-five pounds annually, the rate of diabetes is high—twenty-five of every thousand people, an incidence many times greater than in nations where the intake of sugar and refined starch is low.

Heavy Drinking

Excessive use of alcohol is a critical risk factor because it works against your health in general, and specifically exposes you to other hazards such as injury or even death in a car accident. Alcohol is the single most common cause of traffic accidents. It is a contributing factor in at least half the nation's eighty thousand traffic deaths. The costs of alcohol-related accidents are enormous: $3.5 billion for deaths and $2.4 billion for injuries.

Of course over a long period of time heavy drinking takes its toll on your body. It lowers the body's resistance to disease. It can impair many of the normal functions of the liver. Heavy drinkers also do damage to themselves nutritionally by spending more time draining a glass than eating.

Stress

Stress is unavoidable. In fact there are times when you shouldn't try to avoid it. It can provide zest to everyday life. Dr. Hans Selye, the man most responsible for modern medicine's awareness of stress, says this happy, beneficial pressure actually should be called *eustress*.

The kind most of you want to avoid is the kind that grinds you down, squeezes and stretches you, makes you feel as though you're living inside a pressure cooker. Probably the simplest way to describe any stress is to say it is the nonspecific response of the body to any demand made on it. Surprisingly, this demand can be something either pleasant or unpleasant. Each type can induce the same reactions in our bodies. Stress becomes critical and wearing when the intensity of that demand is too high and it goes on too long.

Each of us has a personal overload threshold just as each of us has an individual pain threshold. What we all share is the fact that ultimately we are all susceptible to the impact of any strong conflict and change. When that conflict or change gets intense enough it can take its toll on our bodies. Although the damaging process is not fully understood, researchers do know that when stress reaches a critical point they can see evidence of it in problems such as depression, ulcers, and heart attacks.

Although you may have a vague notion of the kinds of things that do or do not bring stress to bear on you, it's possible there are a few things you may be overlooking. To help rate your current stress health, take a look at the following list of items put together in the form of a shopping list of stresses called the Life Change Index. It's a way of rating all the stressful events that happened to you in the past year on a 1 to 100 number scale. Researchers have found that most, about three-quarters, of those who score 300 or higher in a year will get ill within that same year.

It's a simple test to take. Read down the list and copy in the far-right column the number rating of any stress that happened to you in the past year. When you finish, add up your total and see what you get. The closer your score edges to 300, the rougher your year has been.

LIFE CHANGE INDEX

Event	Scale of Impact	
Death of Spouse	100	_____
Divorce	73	_____
Marital Separation	65	_____
Jail Term	63	_____
Death of Close Family Member	63	_____
Personal Injury or Illness	53	_____
Marriage	50	_____

Fired From Job .... 47 _____
Marital Reconciliation .... 45 _____
Retirement .... 45 _____
Change in Health of Family Member ...... 44 _____
Pregnancy .... 40 _____
Sex Difficulties .... 39 _____
Gain of New Family Member .... 39 _____
Business Readjustment .... 39 _____
Change in Financial State .... 38 _____
Death of Close Friend .... 37 _____
Change to Different Line of Work .... 36 _____
Change in Number of Arguments with
Spouse .... 35 _____
Mortgage over $40,000 .... 31 _____
Foreclosure of Mortgage or Loan .... 30 _____
Change in Responsibilities at Work .... 29 _____
Son or Daughter Leaving Home .... 29 _____
Trouble with In-Laws .... 29 _____
Outstanding Personal Achievement .... 28 _____
Spouse Begins or Stops Work .... 26 _____
Begin or End School .... 26 _____
Change in Living Conditions .... 25 _____
Revision of Personal Habits .... 24 _____
Trouble with Boss .... 23 _____
Change in Work Hours or Conditions ...... 20 _____
Change in Residence .... 20 _____
Change in Schools .... 20 _____
Change in Recreation .... 19 _____
Change in Church Activities .... 19 _____
Change in Social Activities .... 18 _____
Mortgage or Loan Less than $40,000 .... 17 _____
Change in Sleeping Habits .... 16 _____
Change in Number of Family Get-
Togethers .... 15 _____

Change in Eating Habits .... 15 _____
Vacation .... 13 _____
Christmas (if approaching) .... 12 _____
Minor Violations of the Law .... 11 _____
                              TOTAL   _____

RISK AGE: HOW OLD ARE YOU, REALLY?

All those critical risk factors—smoking, overeating, heavy drinking, stress—and some of the other physical problems they bring age us imperceptibly. For example, although your chronological age may be thirty-five, if you have an elevated cholesterol level, high blood pressure, drink and smoke heavily, you easily have aged yourself another fifteen years. In others words your birth certificate may identify you as someone who is thirty-five but a thorough physical exam would put your life expectancy as being the same as the average fifty-year-old.

This is what I mean by risk age. You have managed to accelerate the aging process and shorten your life expectancy by a life style that is literally wearing you out. Fortunately, it is a process you can stop and even reverse.

"Is there anyone in America today who doesn't know that too much fat, too much salt, too much alcohol, and too many of these things are bad for you?" asked my friend from Los Angeles, pointing to her cigarette. "I know the air in this city is awful and the water tastes funny and I work too hard and should take more time off," she went on, getting more anxious all the time.

"I've given up salt and red meat and rum raisin ice cream. I run every morning and I do yoga once a week. Can't I go on living here—I really love it—and working hard and smoking, if I do everything else in my life according to your self-health magic plan?"

Of course, she knew what the answer to that was going

to be, but she also saw that I would understand—and be sympathetic to what she was asking. Yes, she should stop smoking; yes, she should do something to protect herself against the environmental hazards in her city; yes, she should reduce some of the stresses, in her life; and no, as much as I might like to claim differently, the self-health plan is not magic.

But it's the next best thing.

The plain fact is that by following the self-health plan you can reduce your risk age by five, ten, even fifteen years. If you also manage to kick a heavy smoking habit, you can subtract two more years from your risk age. If you get your high blood pressure down to a normal level, take at least one more year from your risk age. And if you quit a heavy drinking habit, you can further reduce it by another eleven years. As far as your personal health is concerned, you can turn back the clock.

Before you can do anything, you first have to know what your own risk age is now. You do that by filling out the following questionnaire—I promise this is the last one—and you will be more aware of the kinds of hazards to which you subject yourself. It's a simple multiple choice quiz. Simply mark on the line to the right of each question the appropriate number and, when you are finished, add up all the numbers. That total will tell you how old you really are in terms of risk factors.

YOUR RISK AGE PROFILE

Exercise

1. Amount of physical effort expended during the workday: mostly
   a) Heavy physical, walking, housework .. 1
   b) Desk work .... 3 _____
2. Participation in physical activities—(skiing,

golf, swimming, gardening, etc.)
  a) Daily 1
  b) Weekly 3
  c) Seldom .... 5 _____
3. Participation in a vigorous exercise program
  a) Three times weekly 1
  b) Weekly 3
  c) Seldom .... 5 _____
4. Average miles walked or jogged per day
  a) More than one 1
  b) Less than one 3
  c) None .... 5 _____
5. Flights of stairs climbed per day
  a) More than ten 1
  b) Less than ten .... 3 _____

Nutrition

6. Are you overweight?
  a) No 1
  b) Five to nineteen pounds 3
  c) More than twenty pounds .... 5 _____
7. Do you eat a wide variety of foods—something from each of the following five food groups: (1) meat, fish, poultry, dried legumes, eggs, or nuts; (2) milk or milk products; (3) bread or cereals; (4) fruits; (5) vegetables
  a) Each day 1
  b) Three times weekly .... 3 _____

Alcohol

8. Average number of bottles (12 oz.) of beer per week
  a) Zero to seven 1
  b) Eight to fifteen 3

c) More than sixteen................................ 5 _____
9. Average number of hard liquor (1½ oz.) drinks per week
    a) Zero to seven 1
    b) Eight to fifteen 3
    c) More than sixteen................................ 5 _____
10. Average number of glasses (5 oz.) of wine per week
    a) Zero to seven 1
    b) Eight to fifteen 3
    c) More than sixteen................................ 5 _____
11. Total number of drinks per week, including beer, liquor, and wine
    a) Zero to seven 1
    b) Eight to fifteen 3
    c) More than sixteen................................ 5 _____

Drugs

12. Do you take drugs legally?
    a) No 1
    b) Yes.. 3 _____
13. Do you consume alcoholic beverages together with certain drugs (tranquillizers, barbiturates, antihistamines or illegal drugs)?
    a) No 1
    b) Yes.. 5 _____
14. Do you use pain-killers improperly or excessively?
    a) No 1
    b) Yes.. 5 _____

Tobacco

15. Cigarettes smoked per day
    a) None 1

   b) Ten 3
   c) More than ten.............................. 5 _____
16. Cigars smoked per day
   a) None 1
   b) Five 3
   c) More than five .... 5 _____
17. Pipe tobacco pouches per week
   a) None 1
   b) Two 3
   c) More than two .... 5 _____

Personal Health
18. Do you experience periods of depression?
   a) Seldom 1
   b) Occasionally 3
   c) Frequently .... 5 _____
19. Does anxiety interfere with your daily activities?
   a) No 1
   b) Occasionally 3
   c) Frequently .... 5 _____
20. Do you get enough satisfying sleep?
   a) Yes.. 1
   b) No .... 3 _____
21. Are you aware of the causes and dangers of VD?
   a) Yes.. 1
   b) No .... 3 _____
22. Breast self-examination (if not applicable, do not score)
   a) Monthly 1
   b) Occasionally .... 3 _____

Road and Water Safety
23. Mileage per year as driver or passenger

a) Less than ten thousand 1
b) More than ten thousand........................ 3 _____
24. Do you often exceed the speed limit?
    a) No 1
    b) By more than 10 mph. 3
    c) By more than 20 mph. .... 5 _____
25. Do you wear a seat belt?
    a) Always.. 1
    b) Occasionally 3
    c) Never.. 5 _____
26. Do you drive a motorcycle, moped, or snowmobile?
    a) No 1
    b) Yes.. 3 _____
27. If yes to the above, do you always wear a regulation safety helmet? (If not applicable, do not score.)
    a) Yes.. 1
    b) No .... 5 _____
28. Do you ever drive under the influence of alcohol?
    a) Never.. 1
    b) Occasionally .... 5 _____
29. Do you ever drive when your ability may be affected by drugs?
    a) Never.. 1
    b) Occasionally .... 5 _____
30. Are you aware of water safety rules?
    a) Yes.. 1
    b) No .... 3 _____
31. If you participate in water sports or boating, do you wear a life jacket? (If not applicable, do not score.)
    a) Yes.. 1

b) No .... 3 _____

General

32. Average number of hours watching TV per day
    a) Zero to one 1
    b) One to four 3
    c) More than four .... 5 _____

33. Are you familiar with first-aid procedures?
    a) Yes 1
    b) No .... 3 _____

34. Do you ever smoke in bed?
    a) No 1
    b) Occasionally 3
    c) Yes .... 5 _____

TOTAL _____

Now that you've identified and rated the different elements in your risk age, you can see the critical spots in your life style that are making you older than you should be. How do you know how well you did? Match your total score against this risk age scale:

If your total score is:	Then your current risk age is:
45 or lower	Excellent
46–55	Good
56–65	Risky
66 or higher	High Risk

At this point you should have a clearer idea of just how healthy you are, as well as what needs to be adjusted to give you more complete control over your life and health. To help give you even greater control, in the chapters to come you will learn specific self-health techniques you can use in a personal program for achievement, better health, and better looks. As you prepare to begin, you should first glance over the following checklist of life extenders. You may want to refer to it during the first twelve weeks of your own self-health program. At the end of the twelve weeks it's not a bad idea to turn back to this section and see what life extenders you can use more effectively in your self-health plan.

THE LIFE EXTENDERS

The following concepts help you establish the right habits and the right frame of mind to adopt a lifelong habit of fitness and good health. Some of them are things to do; some, things not to do. All are chosen with one goal in mind: if followed consistently, they will enhance and extend your life.

• UNDERSTAND YOUR PHYSICAL SELF: Get to know all you can about your body, its abilities and its limitations, moods, its sensitivities. It is an amazing machine, a beautifully coordinated construction of 206 bones and more than 600 muscles. It has to be used and cared for intelligently if you are going to enjoy all the benefits it can give you.

• UNDERSTAND NUTRITION: You can't expect a body to operate well unless it's fueled well. If you've never gotten around to learning exactly what good nutrition is, now is the time to do so. It is not as complicated or dreary an undertaking as you might think, and ultimately it can only be to your benefit. Even if you think you know everything worth knowing about nutrition, take the time to read the sections that follow on the subject. You may get a few surprises.

• KEEP YOUR BODY ACTIVE: A key part of the self-health program is to develop the habit of exercise, if

28

you don't already have one. Exercise is not only good for your body, keeping it supple and in tone, it is good for the mind. It's a valuable safety valve for releasing the pressures of stress and it does wonders for your self-image.

• WATCH YOUR WEIGHT: As any doctor will tell you the hardest part of any diet is not losing weight, but keeping it off. The effort is worth it. By staying at or close to your ideal weight you are avoiding most of the risk that comes automatically with having too many extra pounds. You have to make sure that your eating style keeps pace with your life style. Otherwise you're going to find those pounds constantly creeping up on you. Fortunately, by following the balanced program of self-health nutrition and exercise, this vigil is much easier and more satisfying than a continuing series of crash diets.

• DISARM YOUR INTERNAL ENVIRONMENT: Do you constantly race against time? Do you work obsessively? You have to take the time to build into your day release valves for all that tension and pressure that you're stopping up within yourself. Exercise, as I've already mentioned, is a good release. And so is whatever else you find useful, whether it's meditation, yoga, or some other peaceful, unwinding activity. Everyone—young, old and in between—needs playtime of some sort. It's the best and most readily available prescription for reducing stress.

• DISARM YOUR PHYSICAL ENVIRONMENT: If you live in or near a major urban area, you are probably acutely aware of how your environment assaults you. There are certain things out of your immediate control—bad air and noise for example—but you can disconnect yourself from some of the corrosive effects of what is around you. You can start by being careful about what you put into your body. Polluting it with bad food, smoke, or too much alcohol only puts your environment more in control of you rather than the other way around. Also, if you become sensitive to your stress limits, you will know when you're approaching the overload point. That is a good time to get away from it all—to purify your system with the fresh air and quiet surroundings that a rural environment offers. Nature is one of the best therapeutic agents available to you.

• AVOID THE DRUG AND ALCOHOL TRAP: Scientists have yet to find a chemical way to unwind that's completely safe. Not only do both drugs and drinks offer you little in the way of genuine relaxation, if they get to be a habit they will turn on you, doing much more harm than good.

• FINALLY, STOP SMOKING: This is easier said than done as anyone who's tried to quit well knows. But if you are sincerely interested in keeping the good health you have and improving on it, the task will be a lot simpler. The self-health program can and will do you good even if you continue smoking, but its benefits will be so much greater if you can get yourself off the nicotine habit.

HOW TO IMPROVE YOUR SCORE

If you're not satisfied with your risk age score you can change it. This is one instance where you can literally reverse the aging process. If you are a forty-year-old, you can reach a risk age of thirty-five in about twelve weeks.

In the pages to come you will be given the basics of this unique revitalizing nutrition and exercise plan and also learn how to customize it to make it work for you. You will plan your own program and suit it to your needs, to your life style. And the results will be immediate. In just one day you will start to change and in twelve weeks you will see this change as you get control of your health and your life. The first step in the program is getting to know your nutritional needs.

2

NUTRITIONAL GOALS FOR THE WHOLE YOU

Most of us are aware of the importance of good nutrition, but many of us do not practice it. Why? The truth is that many of us either know little about basic nutrition or are confused by the constant flurry of health and diet fads about what is good for us and what isn't. Many of us have not been educated in the principles of good nutrition or have not been encouraged to relate proper nutrition to good health. "So much of what we think and do is determined by factors we haven't reflected on or mastered," explains obesity expert Dr. Theodore VanItallie, "such as the nature of our diet, the constant display of advertised temptations. . . ." We are constantly bombarded with commercials and ads for sweets, fast foods, heavily sugared drinks, and snacks. Given this situation, it's hard enough to remember that good nutrition is directly related to a longer, healthier life, much less to find out how to get past all that junk-food noise to the truth.

Fortunately, there is more information than ever

about the relationship between good nutrition and good health and it is being given more attention and publicity than ever before. No longer are advocates of better nutrition dismissed as food faddists and health-food nuts. The evidence is already in that how we eat has a direct bearing on how healthy or sick we are.

Dr. Jesse Marmorston, professor of clinical medicine at the University of Southern California, is the principal investigator on the university's Multiple Risk Factor Intervention Trial (MR FIT) program and has watched the effects of a good diet at work. She has the following to say on the subject of diet and health:

"For the past three years, I have supervised a program involving 5,000 people who have suffered one or more heart attacks or strokes, or who are high risk heart attack candidates. Although the findings of this program are not complete, so far they have shown that the self-health approach—a diet low in fat and high in carbohydrates, plus a well-designed exercise program—has reduced risk factors dramatically in this nationwide program sponsored by the Department of Health, Education and Welfare together with the American Heart Association. Self-health offers a dynamic program that builds and maintains healthy lives."

To get started on this program you first have to raise your nutritional consciousness a little. Take the time to stop and study your eating habits, evaluate them, and, where necessary, change them. Self-health will help you do all this. It will also teach you *what to eat,* in *what proportions,* and *why.*

DIET AND DISEASE

The first step is to answer that last question: why eat nutritionally? There's the general benefit of good health—looking better, feeling better—but there are, doctors have found, some very specific benefits as well. Nutritionists are convinced that each year hundreds of thousands of lives could be improved, extended, and even saved if people were more careful about following a dietary program of complete nutrition.

Diet and Cancer

According to Dr. Gio Gori, deputy director of the National Cancer Institute, 40 percent of cancer cases among men and 60 percent of the cancer cases among women are related to their diet. For example, in studying breast cancer, the most serious cancer risk to women, Dr. Ernest Wynder of the American Health Foundation says that wherever this cancer is found in the world it is associated with a high-fat diet. He also discovered other strong correlations between a low-fiber diet in Western societies and a high rate of cancer of the colon and rectum. These particular cancers are virtually unknown in populations whose diets include a great deal of fiber. Added to these cancer risks is the growing list of chemical additives and preservatives coming under more critical scrutiny as possible cancer-causing agents.

Diet and Heart Disease

Research has pinpointed specific imprudent eating habits which, if eliminated, could decrease significantly the number of casualties from heart disease, the country's number-one killer. The villains are a high-cholesterol diet and obesity. As you have already seen, both are contributing factors to high blood pressure, a prime risk factor in heart disease. In the next *hour* ten thousand men and women in the United States will suffer heart attacks. If they had taken the time to learn a little more about the right diet, the attacks might have been avoided.

Diet and Mental Health

There are close to 20 million Americans who need some kind of mental health care, according to the National Institute of Mental Health. And it is more than likely, say many scientists, that some of these same people who are suffering from problems such as schizophrenia and hyperactivity can be helped by a change in diet. Psychiatrist Michael Lesser of Berkeley, California, has found that almost 70 percent of his patients who have mental problems also suffer from low blood sugar or hypoglycemia. Dr. Abraham Hoffer, a Canadian forensic psychiatrist, has suggested that 70 percent of convicts imprisoned in jails in his province suffer from some form of vitamin deficiency, and their criminal behavior could be explained at least partially by this fact. One San Francisco physician, Dr. Benjamin Feingold, became nationally famous when he discovered that by eliminating foods containing a certain red-dye additive from the diets of hyperactive children, he could reduce their hyperactivity.

Today we know that many so-called mental illnesses and even fatigue can be the result of low blood sugar or deficiencies in niacin, vitamins B-1, B-6, B-12, vitamin C (ascorbic acid), or certain amino acids (proteins). For that reason doctors have found that taking a high potency B-complex vitamin and even a supplemental dose of vitamin C erase many of the body's deficiencies that surface as fatigue or general nervousness.

Although it is not yet clear exactly why certain vitamins have this effect on our mental health, it shouldn't be surprising to see that the nutritional chemistry of our diets works on the mind. The brain, after all, is part of the body and as such has to have a certain balanced chemistry to work normally. Disrupt this and you disrupt many of its functions. Since the brain houses our thoughts and emotions and is the coordinator for our senses, a chemically imbalanced brain could express itself in disordered thoughts, emotional upsets, and even disturbed sensory perceptions.

FUEL FOR YOUR ECOSYSTEM

To protect yourself from these dietary upsets, you need the right balance of six basic food components in your diet. They are: proteins, carbohydrates, fats, fiber, minerals, and vitamins. Before you start learning what that right balance is, you should have at least a general idea of what each component does.

Protein   2084170

Everyone seems to be talking about protein these days: will there be enough in the twenty-first century? Do we need more? Less? Do we need it at all? Although the answers to the first three questions are debated, there's no doubt about the answer to the last one. We absolutely, positively need protein for the most basic reasons. Protein is the body's chief building block. It's also the second most abundant substance in the body. It maintains body tissue, is essential to building cells and keeping them alive, and it develops muscle, skin, nails, hair, and internal organs. It is used to build the enzymes controlling the chemical reactions that go on inside your body every second of your life. Finally, it is a necessary part of your body's immune system and is a prime ingredient of the hormones that regulate metabolism.

The body needs large amounts of protein whenever it has to build new tissue quickly: during pregnancy, during a child's growing years, and when protein is lost because of an injury, an infection, or surgery. Every daily diet needs some protein, simply because your body can store very little of it. If you eat large amounts of protein and don't use it all, that excess protein will become fat. One important thing to remember is that protein calories are no less fattening than carbohydrate calories or calories from fats. For that reason you have to be as careful about protein consumption as any other food component.

All food proteins are made of carbon, hydrogen, oxygen, nitrogen, and small quantities of other elements such as phosphorous and iron. During digestion your body breaks down large protein molecules into simpler units called amino acids. These compounds are necessary for turning food protein into human protein. Your body needs approximately twenty-two of these amino acids to make its own protein. Many of these it can produce itself, but there are eight essential amino acids that it cannot make. These have to be gotten directly from your food.

Food that contains these eight essential amino acids are grouped under the heading of complete protein. Meats, fish, fowl, and most dairy products fall into the complete protein category. Incomplete proteins, on the other hand, are those that either lack or are low in any of the eight essential amino acids. Most vegetables, fruits, and cereals are considered incomplete proteins. Being aware of the differences between the two proteins is essential to planning the right diet for you. For example a typical (700 calories) meal with a good balance of both types of proteins would be:

- Roast chicken
- Salad—tomatoes, spinach
- Dessert—pineapple boat (pineapple, strawberries, sliced banana)
- Drink—fruit juice of choice

This is only a sample menu drawn up to give you an idea of what a typical well-balanced protein meal would be like. (In Chapter Four you'll find a more thorough discussion of the well-balanced diet complete with suggested menus.) This meal also has a good balance of carbohydrates as well. In general, nutritional research has found that you, assuming you're the average adult, should be getting 12 percent of your daily caloric needs from the protein in your diet.

Later you will learn how to gauge both your caloric need and protein intake, but for now, if you are looking for a good diet supplement that is an ideal source of protein, make a note to buy some bee pollen. Available in most health food stores, this is a natural food source that has all the water-soluble vitamins, essential minerals, and all twenty-two amino acids in ideal proportions for human consumption. Bee pollen is used in treating colitis, high blood pressure, and various allergies. It helps flush from your circulatory system fat-forming and oxygen-robbing impurities and, taken regularly, helps you resist the wear and tear of stress. It also will give you more stamina and help speed your recovery from illness. It is the richest natural source of your protein needs known, and a diet supplement you should consider.

Carbohydrates

You've probably seen carbohydrates named as the food villain in many fad diets. This is misleading because carbohydrates are no more fattening than fats or proteins. Excess calories from any of the food groups will always mean excess weight. You need carbohydrates for a healthy diet. They are the most common and most efficient source of energy available to your body. After you eat foods rich in carbohydrates your digestive system changes the carbohydrates into glucose, a natural energy source needed by all the tissues of your body.

Carbohydrates are simple sugars or compound sugars that can be broken down into simple sugars. They come under a variety of names in a variety of foods. Fructose, for example, is the name for the natural sugar found in fruit, and lactose is the name for the natural sugar in milk. Generally, carbohydrates exist in three different forms:

Single-sugar units: Also called monosaccharides, they are the most common example of the natural sugar glucose found in our bloodstream.

Two-sugar units: Also known as disaccharides, they are typically the sugars found in vegetables. These are called sucrose.

Multiple-sugar units: These are called polysaccharides and are found as starch in vegetables such as potatoes.

Nutritionists say that the average adult should make sure that carbohydrates make up 58 percent of his or her daily diet. As you will see in the next chapter, it is also important that you choose the correct carbohydrates to satisfy this requirement.

Fats

Fats—or rather the elimination of them—have been the target of nearly as many diet taboos as carbohydrates. A diet without fats, however, is an incomplete one. Fats are necessary for proper growth, healthy skin, and they carry essential vitamins such as A, D, E, and K. Like carbohydrates they are also rich sources of energy for your body. They are absolutely essential for good nutrition.

Fats are generally described as being saturated or unsaturated. This refers to the basic structure of fatty acids, prime ingredients in fats. Each fatty acid is made up of a series of carbon atoms joined together like links on a chain.

Each carbon atom is capable of attracting to it and holding a certain number of hydrogen atoms. A fatty acid where the carbon atoms are all holding their limits is called a *saturated* fat. Sometimes it happens that in this atomic chain two adjacent carbon atoms have no hydrogen atoms attached to them and they form a double bond between them. When this happens, the result is called an *unsaturated* fat. Saturated and unsaturated fats do not exist in pure forms in nature. Most fatty foods are mixtures of the two, although as a rule animal fats tend to be highly saturated while liquid vegetable oils, such as corn oils, are more unsaturated.

For dietary reasons the saturated fats are the ones that deserve your concern. Research indicates that a diet high in saturated fats may cause an increase in blood levels of cholesterol which in turn is a risk factor in heart disease. Doctors found, for example, that white middle-aged American men (thirty to fifty-nine) with high cholesterol levels (250 to 299 milligrams) also had twice as many heart attacks as men the same age but with lower (175–249 milligrams) cholesterol levels. Doctors also suspect that high-fat diets may be implicated in breast cancer. That particular cancer, they found, is rare among women in Japan but it has been known to be higher among Japanese immigrants to the United States after they switch to the typically high-fat American diet.

Still, you need fats. Nutritionists say 30 percent of your daily caloric intake should come from fats. The trick is picking the right ones.

Fiber

For years fiber was one of the more overlooked food components. Fortunately, as a result of dietary discoveries in recent years, that has changed. Studies have found that the right amount of fiber in your diet is especially effective as a safeguard against diseases of the lower intestine: cancer of the colon, colitis or inflammation of the large bowel, and another painful form of intestinal inflammation, diverticulitis. These ailments rarely occur among people whose diet is high in fiber and low in processed foods.

Fiber is made of cellulose and other substances that make up the cell walls and structural formations in plants. Celery, bran, and apple skins are all high-fiber foods. Fiber is unique among the food components because it has no nutritional value. It is not broken down by our digestive systems, but it does stimulate the normal action of the intestines and help eliminate waste products. These last two features make it a valuable addition to your diet.

Minerals

Having the right amount of minerals in your body can literally be a matter of life and death. It would be hard to think of a bodily need or function that wasn't dependent on minerals. Totaling about 4 percent of your body weight, minerals come from your food alone. Your body cannot produce them. Without minerals you would not grow, your nervous system would shut down, you could bleed to death from a small cut on your finger—to give you an idea of how important they are.

You need different amounts of different minerals, sometimes in minute quantities. Whatever the amounts, you also need fresh supplies constantly. Some minerals are absorbed into your body and held, while others are used and discarded. They are only partially absorbed from the mineral-rich foods you may eat, and some are absorbed more easily than others. You will find out later how to get the right amount of mineral-rich foods in your diet. For now this brief descriptive list should give you some idea of the range of bodily needs minerals serve.

• *Calcium* is the mineral which, as everyone probably already knows from a famous ad campaign, "builds strong bones and teeth." It is especially important for bone development and growth. Everyone needs it, of course, but growing children, pregnant women, and older people need it the most. Calcium is also necessary, say doctors, for the normal functioning of muscles and nerves. Leafy vegetables and especially dairy products are rich in this basic mineral.

• *Copper* is needed in only small amounts in your body primarily for its role in manufacturing hemoglobin, the red-blood-cell pigment that carries oxygen in your bloodstream.

• *Iodine* is absolutely necessary for the normal functioning of your thyroid gland. Without it you could not produce thyroid hormones. Seafood and iodized salt are probably the most common sources of this mineral.

• *Iron* is another mineral needed for making hemoglobin and is an ingredient in many body enzymes. Women who are menstruating or pregnant or who are breast-feeding especially need this mineral and often take dietary iron supplements in addition to getting it from ordinary food sources such as meat and eggs.

• *Magnesium* together with calcium is important to good teeth and bones but it is also a vital ingredient in muscle contractions. Foods high in this mineral include: peanuts, beans, whole grains, and dairy products.

• *Phosphorous* together with calcium and magnesium is the other mineral most important for having sound bones and teeth. Your kidneys and nervous system also need this to function properly. One of the more accessible minerals—it's found in just about every food from eggs to seafood—phosphorous is seldom in short supply in our diet.

• *Zinc* is needed in tiny amounts in the body but it still

plays an important part in your metabolism. Many of your body's enzymes need zinc and there is also evidence that this mineral is vital to regulation of the action of your pancreas and control of your body's cholesterol level.

Vitamins

Vitamins and minerals often work closely together helping your body get and use food energy, building up tissue, and serving as the raw material for needed body chemicals. Unlike minerals, which are *in* organic compounds, vitamins *are* organic compounds or chemicals. Vitamins are either fat-soluble—that is, they need the presence of fat to be absorbed into your body—or they are water-soluble, which means they dissolve in water and are more easily absorbed into your body. Given here in alphabetical order are the more important ones.

• *Vitamin A* is a fat-soluble vitamin especially important for normal growth, healthy skin, and keeping the body's mucous membranes moist. People deficient in this vitamin sometimes suffer from "night blindness," difficulty adjusting the eyes to the dark after gazing at a bright light; dry skin; slowed growth in skin and nerve tissue; and an increased susceptibility to infections of the skin, ears, sinuses, lungs, bladder, and digestive tract. Those who have too much of this vitamin may suffer from loss of hair and pains in the joints. It can be extremely toxic in large doses. It comes from carotene, a substance commonly found in carrots and other plants such as spinach and broccoli and in liver, eggs, and dairy products.

• *Vitamin B*, actually a vitamin group that falls under the general name of vitamin B-complex, is a water-soluble vitamin. Included under the vitamin B-complex grouping are: thiamin or B-1; riboflavin or B-2; niacin or B-3; pyridoxine or B-6; B-12; biotin; folic acid; inositol; pantothenic acid; PABA; and choline. As far as your brain is concerned, this is the single most important vitamin group. It is absolutely necessary for the smooth functioning of your brain and nervous system. If you are deficient in a B-complex vitamin, you could be plagued with everything from a sluggish brain and nervous system, depression and hallucinations to beriberi and vision problems. Foods such as whole grain cereals, green vegetables, legumes, brewer's yeast, and milk and eggs are rich in B-complex.

Two of the B-complex group worth discussing separately are the vitamins PABA (for para-aminobenzoic acid) and choline. Technically a vitamin within a vitamin, PABA helps stimulate intestinal bacteria necessary for your digestion and is vital to skin and hair health. It also plays a big part in the working of your body's enzymes. In the form of a cream, PABA is also a safe and effective suntan lotion. In foods you will find it in wheat germ, liver, yeast, and molasses.

Choline is important to your body because it helps you dissolve the fats and cholesterol in your bloodstream and is an important element in your body's manufacture of thyroid hormones. Many of the B-complex foods—liver, wheat germ, yeast and egg yolk—are rich in it.

• *Vitamin C* is a water-soluble vitamin that researchers know protects the body against infection and acts as a valuable antistress substance as well. Also known by its chemical name of *ascorbic acid*, this vitamin is found most plentifully in citrus fruits but is also present in vegetables such as tomatoes and broccoli.

• *Vitamin D* is a fat-soluble vitamin unique in that it comes naturally from two places: sunlight and fish oils such as cod liver oil. It is absolutely necessary for normal bone growth and good teeth. Too little of this vitamin can result in bone deformities, the childhood disease of rickets being a good example. Too much vitamin D could be toxic, causing a buildup of calcium in the blood vessels and organs of the body. The action of sunlight on human skin oils produces vitamin D in the body. You can also add the vitamin to your diet by drinking vitamin D-enriched milk.

• *Vitamin E* is a fat-soluble vitamin sometimes called the purifying vitamin because it offers protection against many of the environmental poisons in our air, water, and food. It brings nourishment to the cells of your body, helps strengthen capillary walls, and protects oxygen-carrying red cells from toxins. It also unites with oxygen and holds it in a pure form so that more of the gas is absorbed into the blood and delivered to the rest of the body. This helps circulation and promotes vitality. Researchers have found that this vitamin has helped lower blood cholesterol by preventing fat deposits, and it also seems to raise the body's natural resistance to infection. One of the richest sources of this vitamin is wheat germ, but it is also found in liver, beans, peas, and leafy green vegetables.

• *Vitamin K* is another fat-soluble vitamin essential to the blood's ability to clot. Without this vitamin you could be susceptible to internal bleeding and even hemorrhaging. Most foods such as leafy green vegetables, potatoes, bran, and tomatoes are rich in this necessary vitamin, as are yogurt and blackstrap molasses.

One other nutrient you might want to include in your diet is a natural substance called ribonucleic acid, better known as RNA. It's a natural food substance found most commonly in yeast, which is 6 percent RNA, and research indicates that it is valuable in retarding some of the effects of aging, specifically senility. Sometimes nicknamed the "memory molecule," RNA has been thought to be a prime ingredient in the brain's complicated biochemical mechanism of memory and learning. Researchers who have given the substance, extracted from yeast, to senile patients have seen improvement in their condition. It also seems to have other benefits. It is a nutrient for the skin, improving tone and appearance, and in general seems to be a revitalizer.

With a standard daily dose of two to ten grams of RNA you should get some of its benefits. It is available in many health-food stores but before you buy it and use it there are a few things to keep in mind. First, never buy an RNA substance that has less than a 12 percent concentration of the acid. Anything with a lower concentration than this is just overpriced yeast. Second, RNA *is* an acid and it may upset your stomach. You can get around that problem by taking a little baking soda with it. Finally, RNA raises the level of uric acid in your system. Ordinarily this is no problem, but if you are susceptible to gout, you already have a naturally high uric-acid level and should leave this nutrient out of your diet.

PUTTING IT ALL TOGETHER

Knowing what these various food components do for your body is only part of your nutritional education. You also have to know how to organize them into a complete daily dietary program that will satisfy your body's needs and at the same time help you avoid many of the risk factors that come with a lopsided intake of certain foods.

This may sound complicated. On the one hand, you have to make sure you get the right daily intake of proteins, carbohydrates, fats, fiber, minerals, and vitamins from your meals. On the other hand, you have to be concerned about keeping fats and cholesterol in your system down to an acceptable level, and you have to keep your caloric intake fixed at a point where you use every calorie you eat and don't end up gaining excess weight.

Fortunately it is not at all difficult if you follow the self-health diet. It's important to stress here that, although it can help you lose weight, this is not primarily a weight-losing diet. It is a lifelong nutritional blueprint you can use to:

- reduce your intake of fats and cholesterol
- reduce your intake of risky foods, those that have been implicated in various diseases
- help get your weight down, if that is necessary, to a healthy normal level and keep it there
- help you automatically use the right combinations of foods in your daily meals by giving you the best sources of all six food components

Now that you've learned why your body needs what it feeds from foods, the next step is to find the best foods to satisfy these needs.

3

THE SELF-HEALTH FOODS

The last hundred years of our civilization has been marked by tremendous advances in every aspect of modern life but one—the length of human life itself. With all of the medical and scientific expertise, all the technological wizardry at our disposal, we have still managed to extend the average life span by only about three years. The reason is that for every medical step forward we've made over the years, we as a country have also managed to take a nutritional step back. Although science and medicine have done their part toward stretching our life spans by being able to detect, treat, and cure more human ailments than ever before, we have managed to cancel out some of that progress by giving them more serious ailments to treat. This is largely because we are so careless about our health habits in general and our diet in particular. And the carelessness is spreading. Wherever the so-called Standard American Diet (SAD) has been adopted, usually in affluent countries such as ours, in its wake have come a high and rising rate of heart disease, hypertension, diabetes, and cancer of the breast, stomach, and colon.

For years we've been waiting for medicine and technology to do what we've had in our power all along: extend our life spans. It's really very easy. The key is picking a diet that will satisfy all your nutritional needs and spare you many of the risk factors now built into the sad SAD. This is the self-health diet.

ORIGINS OF THE DIET

Doctors have known or at least suspected for years that there was a direct relation between diet and some of the killer diseases that afflict us. One authority who has proved this to his satisfaction is Dr. Kaare Norum of the University of Oslo. He wanted to know what could be done to eliminate this diet-disease link. To find out he drew up a lengthy questionnaire and sent to an international elite of experts, two hundred scientists in twenty-three countries around the world. He had been investigating the connection between disease, diet, and various environmental factors and he wanted to sound out other experts on what could be done about these health factors, especially nutrition. The results of his survey made up a special issue of the *Journal of the Norwegian Medical Association.*

Included in the survey was a list of dietary priorities that outlined what is today the essential self-health nutritional program. Very simply, the report advised that if you wished to look better, feel better, and live longer, and you were eating the standard diet of affluent societies such as the Standard American Diet, your diet should have:

- fewer calories
- less total fat

- less saturated fat
- more polyunsaturated fat
- less cholesterol
- less salt
- less sugar
- more fiber
- more carbohydrates

Shortly after Dr. Norum published his findings, the need for greater nutritional awareness was officially recognized in the United States. The Select Committee on Nutrition and Human Needs of the United States Senate held weeks of hearings covering in exhaustive detail many of the same issues discussed in Dr. Norum's report. Scientists and doctors from all over the world participated, contributing their expertise and opinion to this forum on nutrition. Among the findings on nutrition that were presented, confirmed, and accepted at the hearings were Dr. Norum's recommendations about what had to be changed in the modern diet to make it less dangerous and more completely nutritious.

The result of weeks of testimony was an eight-volume collection of observations and conclusions concerning the state of the diet in the United States. The most succinct summation of those conclusions was written by Senator George McGovern, one of the committee's principle investigators, in a foreword to the published record of the hearings. "The simple fact is that our diets have changed radically within the last fifty years with great and often harmful effect on our health," he wrote. "These dietary changes represent as great a threat to public health as smoking. Too much fat, too much sugar, can be and are linked directly to heart disease, cancer, obesity, and stroke, among other killer diseases. In all, six of the ten leading causes of death in the United States have been linked to our diet."

It was a grim way to state what was and is a hopeful message: if you don't like your health, you can change it all by yourself. As a guide to what is needed to be done to improve our diets, the committee drew up a set of dietary goals for the United States which essentially follow Dr. Norum's guidelines. They had mapped out a diet for the twenty-first century. Breaking down the foods you eat into the three main calorie providers—fats, proteins, and carbohydrates—the following chart shows you exactly what changes they recommended.

DIETARY GOALS FOR THE UNITED STATES

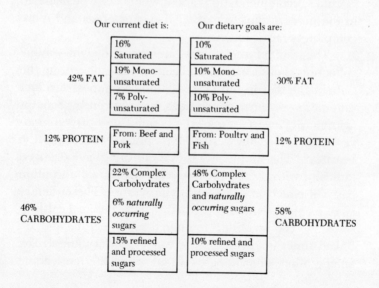

	Our current diet is:	Our dietary goals are:	
42% FAT	16% Saturated 19% Mono-unsaturated 7% Poly-unsaturated	10% Saturated 10% Mono-unsaturated 10% Poly-unsaturated	30% FAT
12% PROTEIN	From: Beef and Pork	From: Poultry and Fish	12% PROTEIN
46% CARBOHYDRATES	22% Complex Carbohydrates 6% *naturally occurring* sugars 15% refined and processed sugars	48% Complex Carbohydrates and *naturally occurring* sugars 10% refined and processed sugars	58% CARBOHYDRATES

The self-health diet has adopted these goals and gives you the techniques to make the dietary shift safely and easily. All these percentages refer to your daily caloric needs from food and nonalcoholic beverages. There are a few terms in this chart that may need a little explanation:

Monounsaturated fats are in a sense neutral fats. They have no apparent effect on blood-cholesterol levels.

Polyunsaturated fats tend to decrease the level of cholesterol in your blood. Complex carbohydrates are those commonly found in fruits and vegetables while "naturally occurring" sugars simply refers to sugars indigenous to foods such as the fructose in fruits. A Bavarian chocolate cake does not have naturally occurring sugar, as much as you might like to think it does. It has sugars in it which are either refined (cane and beet sugar) or processed (as in corn syrup, molasses, and honey).

Without looking too hard, you can see the outline of Dr. Norum's recommendations at work here. This chapter's plan is to help you put those recommendations into action. The way it will do this is by moderate but permanent changes in your diet. Unlike those fad, lose-a-pound-an-hour diets, this is not a two- or three-week starvation binge. This diet is designed to serve you for the rest of your life, not just for the next few weeks. Its ultimate goal is to get you feeling better and living longer. To do this you may have to change some of your long-standing eating habits, but the changes will not commit you to a life of constant self-denial. Most likely you simply will have to cut down a little on some of your favorite dishes or, if you are really a nutritional outlaw, be much more frugal with one or two.

WHO SHOULD FOLLOW THE SELF-HEALTH DIET?

The types of foods recommended in this chapter are suitable for most people from children to adults of all ages. They are all important, necessary elements of any healthy diet. You should note that the *amounts* of foods specified are those recommended for the average healthy *adult*.

CAUTION

The self-health diet is designed for the general population and for average nutritional needs. Of course during different stages of growing up—in infancy, childhood and adolescence—these needs vary. But special needs also occur in adulthood if you are pregnant or are a nursing mother or if you have a diagnosed physical or mental ailment. In these instances the types and amounts of foods you eat should be approved by a physician. If you have any doubt about the appropriateness of the self-health diet for you, consult your doctor. If you are in sound health, the chances are that he or she will not only approve your choice of diet but applaud your decision.

A Word About Salt, Fats, and Cholesterol

Hypertension is a degenerative disease strongly linked to high salt intake. In parts of northern Japan, where large amounts of salt are used in the daily diet, the population has the highest incidence of hypertension in the world. In the United States, where salt is added to most foods despite the fact that many foods contain adequate amounts of natural salt, hypertension is also a serious health problem. But it can be controlled by reducing salt intake.

Just a glance at the dietary goals outlined on page 50 tells you where the most drastic change in your diet will be: fats in foods. If you're eating the typical American diet, you may be in danger of a typical American risk factor, namely, high cholesterol and the increased risk of heart disease that comes with it. To minimize this danger the self-health diet makes a two-part change in your diet. The first is simply to lower your saturated-fat intake. The second is to depend more on polyunsaturated fats for your nutritional needs.

The goal of the diet is to cut down, not to eliminate, cholesterol. You couldn't eliminate it even if you tried. And even if you could, you shouldn't. Your body needs this waxy substance for a variety of processes including manufacturing sex hormones and vitamin D. You always have to have a certain amount in your system for good health.

As you have already seen, the danger comes from having too much. If you eat too many cholesterol-rich foods, the surplus can end up in your blood vessels lining your artery walls with fatty deposits. In time these deposits can build up, narrowing your blood vessels and restricting your blood supply. Blood supplies can be totally cut off to parts of your body this way. When arteries supplying blood to the heart muscle become clogged with fatty deposits the result can be a heart attack.

Arteriosclerosis can develop early in life—it has been found in males in their late teens—and it is an extremely common condition. Not everyone is in danger of it. Some people can have a mild form of it all their lives and never succumb to any of its dangers while in others the disease seems to take hold and worsen rapidly, making them high-risk heart patients.

Why there is this difference is not entirely clear. Some people just seem to inherit a predisposition to the disease. Doctors also know that other factors—excess weight, heavy smoking and drinking, too little exercise, high blood pressure, diabetes—as well as high blood cholesterol aggravate arteriosclerosis.

Fortunately there is much encouraging evidence that taking the time to check or eliminate the risk factors for this ailment can reduce the risk of heart disease. And of course part of this preventive maintenance includes paying close attention to your cholesterol intake.

You get your cholesterol two ways. Some is manufactured inside your body. The liver, for example, is a cholesterol factory. Some comes directly from your food—shrimp, egg yolks, and organ meats are extremely high in this substance. (Plant foods such as fruits, vegetables, grains, cereals and nuts have none. For these reasons you will find much tighter restrictions on cholesterol-rich foods and many fewer restrictions on the others.

Also on the restricted list are saturated fats because they tend to raise the level of cholesterol in the blood. You can get high doses of saturated fat from animal fats and dairy products. Beef, lamb, pork, ham, butter, cream, whole milk, and cheeses made from cream and whole milk are all rich in saturated fats.

Vegetable oil can also be high in saturated fats if it has been hydrogenated or hardened. One of the properties that distinguishes oils from fats is that fats harden at room temperature, while oils stay liquid. Oils can be made to be more like fats through hydrogenation. This is done partially to some of the oils—corn, soybean, and cotton—used in margarines to make them seem more like butter. The more an oil is hydrogenated the harder it gets and the more it resembles a saturated fat. A completely hydrogenated oil is, as far as your body is concerned, the same as saturated fat.

There are also vegetable oils which are naturally high in saturated fats. This group includes coconut oil, cocoa butter, and palm oil, which is often used in factory-made cookies, pie filling, and nondairy cream substitutes.

Polyunsaturated Fats

Since a diet high in saturated fats may increase your

cholesterol level, the self-health program emphasizes foods high in polyunsaturated fats, which tend to lower the level of cholesterol in the blood by helping the body rid itself of excess, newly formed cholesterol. For that reason you will find margarines, which contain only partially hydrogenated oils, on the approved list. They offer the bonus of polyunsaturates absent in butter. Also recommended because of their high level of polyunsaturates are corn, cottonseed, safflower, sesame seed, sunflower seed, and soybean oils. Your daily intake of the fats and oils used in cooking, salads, and flavoring should draw heavily on the polyunsaturated vegetable oils and margarines as part of your continuing cholesterol watch.

Those Forgotten Fats

To heighten your sensitivity to fats in your diet, take a look at this breakdown of foods. All of them provide you with some of your daily caloric needs. The substance in them that gives you those calories varies from food to food. In some cases all or most of the calories are fat calories, which should give you some idea of the concentration of digestible fat in those foods. Take time to read through the list. Some of the groupings may surprise you.

PERCENTAGES OF FAT CALORIES IN FOODS

1. Foods that are over 50 percent fat calories include:

Hot dogs
Pork lunch meats
Ground beef
Pork loin and butt

Tongue
Salmon or tuna packed in oil
Eggs
Cream cheese, most cheeses, and cheese spreads
Peanuts and peanut butter

2. Foods that are 50 percent fat calories include:

Chicken—roasted, flesh and skin
Beef—porterhouse, t-bone, round rump, lean ground,
     kidney
Pork—fresh and cured ham and shoulder
Lamb—shoulder, rib
Salmon—red sockeye, canned
Whole milk
Ice cream
Cream-cheese or peanut-butter sandwich

3. Foods that are 40 percent fat calories are:

Beef—sirloin, flank, and heart
Pork—heart, kidney
Lamb—leg, loin
Turkey—flesh and skin, dark meat
Creamed cottage cheese
Beef lunch-meat or cheese-spread sandwich

4. Foods that are 30 percent fat calories are:

Chicken—broiled light meat without the skin

Beef—heel or round, pot roast
Liver—pork, chicken, lamb, beef
Fish—bass, pink salmon

5. Foods that are 20 percent fat calories include:

Skim milk
Uncreamed cottage cheese
Most breakfast cereals (except granola)

Self-Health: the Key Foods

Now that you have some idea of what you should be looking for in foods, you're probably wondering, like everyone else who opens the morning newspaper and finds yet another food or food additive added to the list of carcinogens, what *can* I eat? You will get a meal-by-meal breakdown in the next chapter, but as a general rule the bulk of your self-health diet will come from a broad but carefully chosen list of foods. To help you pick through the selection on your supermarket shelf, I've worked up what is essentially a guide to self-health foods. There are no strange foods or weird regimens you have to follow with the self-health diet. You most likely eat many of the foods included in the diet. Adjusting to the diet is simply a matter of eating more of one type of food and less of another. Once you get into the habit of thinking more nutritionally about what you eat, you'll probably find yourself instinctively eating this way.

Polyunsaturated Fats and Oils

These are the first foods that have to surface in your food

awareness. On the average you need anywhere from two to four tablespoons (depending on your calorie needs) of these every day in the form of either salad dressing, cooking oils, or margarine. If you use diet margarines you should know that they are low in calories because they are low in fats. For that reason you will need about twice as much diet margarine to supply the polyunsaturates contained in a portion of regular margarine.

Recommended as your daily source of needed fats and oils are:

- High polyunsaturated vegetable oils: corn oil, cottonseed oil, safflower oil, sesame seed oil, soybean oil, and sunflower seed oil.
- Margarines, liquid oil shortenings, salad dressings, and mayonnaise containing those vegetable oils. Make sure to check the ingredients listing for these.

Not recommended as your prime source of fats and oils are solid fats and shortenings such as butter, lard, salt pork fat, completely hydrogenated margarines, vegetable shortenings, and products containing coconut oil. Use these sparingly or, even better, not at all. Peanut oil and olive oil can be used occasionally for their flavor value, but don't depend on them for any nutritional value. They are too low in polyunsaturates to take the place of the approved oils.

Meat

Next on your food-awareness priorities list are meats and meat substitutes, poultry and fish. Following the self-health goal of deemphasizing fats it should come as no surprise to you that the foods most recommended in these categories are:

- poultry—chicken or turkey

- fish—just about all (except the ones packed in oil)
- meat—veal

These should make up the main course in most of your big meals every week. You don't need other kinds of meats although you sometimes may feel otherwise. For those times when you crave beef, or pork, for example, make an effort to choose lean ground meats and lean cuts in general. The chart of saturated fats on page 77 should be a guide. Get in the habit of cutting away excess fat before you bake, broil, or roast. Better yet, make stews with your meat so you can skim off the fats that seep out in the cooking process.

If your dietary ambitions take you in the other direction, toward the elimination of meat from some of your meals, you can turn to these meat substitutes: kidney beans, baked beans, chick peas (garbanzos), split peas, and lima beans. They are all high in vegetable protein and make good occasional substitutes.

On the other hand, use sparingly or avoid completely:

- Poultry: duck or goose—high-fat animals
- Seafood: shrimp, since it is moderately high in cholesterol. You should limit yourself to no more than a four-ounce serving once a week to be eaten in place of meat at that meal.
- Meat: most heavily marbled and fatty meats, which would include some of the higher grades of beef, fatty hamburger, spareribs, mutton, sausages, hot dogs, luncheon meats, and bacon.
- Organ meats: kidney, heart, sweetbreads, and liver—because they are high in cholesterol. Because liver is also rich in vitamins and iron, it is a valuable food source. But eat it sparingly, no more than one four-ounce portion per week.

Fruits and Vegetables

Often overlooked or forgotten as parts of a diet, fruits and vegetables are high-nutrition, no-fat foods that should be included in every meal. They can be eaten as snacks, in salads, as desserts, or even as main courses. They are generally underrated foods and yet are some of your best sources of the recommended daily allowances of vitamins A and C. As you prepare a big meal:

- One serving should be a vitamin A food: broccoli, carrots, chard, chicory, kale, peas, rutabagas, spinach, string beans, sweet potatoes, yams, watercress, winter squash, yellow corn, greens such as beet, collard, dandelion, and turnip, or fruits such as apricots, cantaloupe, mango, or papaya. Yellow fruits and vegetables and dark green leafy vegetables are the best sources for this vitamin.
- One serving should be a vitamin C food: cabbage, raw tomatoes, berries, grapefruit or grapefruit juice, melon, oranges or orange juice, strawberries, or tangerines.

If you are worried about your calories you may substitute some other vegetables for potatoes, corn, and lima beans, which tend to be high-calorie.

Bread and Cereals

Probably the best way to get the kind of bread you want is to do what your ancestors did—bake it. That way you can be sure of getting the right ingredients and the right nutritional benefits. Since you may not have the time to bake, the only other option is to sort through those plastic wrapped loaves of spongy bread piled up in the supermarket and pick out the most nutritious kind. Bread is an important food to think about because it gives you iron and many of your B vitamins. Just be sure when buying bread to read the list of ingredients. If it is white bread, for example, it should be made with enriched flour and a minimum of saturated fats. Ideally, whatever bread you choose should be made from whole grain flour and polyunsaturates.

If a bread meets these standards, almost any type—white enriched, whole wheat, French, Italian, oatmeal, pumpernickel or rye—will do. There are nutritionists who say that whole wheat is more nutritious than the white enriched. Just on the basis of taste, whole wheat is the better choice.

Equally nutritious ways to satisfy bread cravings are English muffins, homemade biscuits, muffins, and griddle cakes that have one of the approved liquid oil shortenings as an ingredient.

Pasta in the form of spaghetti, macaroni, and noodles (but not egg noodles) is also a well-balanced nutritional source, as is rice, especially wild rice and brown rice.

Finally, when it comes to choosing a cereal you should look for one with whole grains and little or no refined sugar. Hot cereals such as oatmeal and farina satisfy this criterion very well, but you'll have to read the ingredients on the side of the box to get an idea of what's in cold cereals. By law, manufacturers must list the ingredients in the order of quantity. The more there is of a substance the closer is will be to the head of the list. If sugar is one of the first ingredients on the side of the box, then the cereal probably has more in it than you need or want.

Foods in the bread and cereal category that you should *avoid or use sparingly* include most commercially made biscuits, muffins, doughnuts, sweet rolls, butter rolls, crackers, egg bread, and commercial mixes with dried egg and whole milk already in them. Read those ingredients lists to make sure.

Dairy and Egg Products

Because of their high fat content, milk and egg products cannot be eaten as freely as, say, most of the vegetables. But this does not mean you must resign yourself to a life without ice cream or your favorite omelet. You just have to use a little more restraint in your milk and egg consumption.

In general if you have a craving for dairy foods try one from this recommended list:

- Milk: stick with fortified skim, or non-fat, milk or fortified low-fat milk powder. Make sure the label on the container specifically says the milk is fortified with vitamins A and D. The word "fortified" alone is not enough. Also in the recommended milk category are buttermilk, cocoa, and yogurt, all made from skimmed milk, as well as canned evaporated skim milk itself.
- Cheeses: you have a good selection of cheese products made with skim or partially skim milk. They include cottage cheese (creamed or, preferably, uncreamed), farmer's cheese, baker's cheese, hoop cheese, and mozzarella.

All of these products are relatively low-fat and for that reason more generously tolerated in the self-health diet. Because they are so fatty, the following dairy and egg products should be *avoided or used sparingly*:

- Whole milk products: chocolate milk, canned or regular whole milk, all creams, half and half, and ice cream.
- Any cheeses made from cream or whole milk.
- Butter
- Eggs: limit yourself to three egg yolks per week. This includes any eggs used as ingredients in foods

such as cake mixes or sauces that use egg yolks in them.

This may mean fewer omelets and milk shakes, but you can probably make up most of your restricted food cravings with selections from the recommended list.

As you can see from reading through these tallies of recommended and restricted foods, the self-health approach to eating does not require monastic discipline and self-denial, just a little more awareness of what you are putting into your body. It's a safe and sane eating program that uses familiar, readily available foods. Part of the beauty of it is that most of the time you are not giving up things so much as substituting foods that are healthier and more nutritious but no less tasty. Just to give some idea of how it can work, here's a quick check list of foods that you may now include in your diet and some self-health substitutes:

If your diet now includes:	*Instead try:*
red meats	poultry and fish
canned vegetables	fresh vegetables
white rice	wild or brown rice; bean
butter	sprouts
ice cream	unsalted margarine, sour
whole milk	cream
soft drinks	fruit ice
sugar	skim milk
salt	fruit juice
sugared cereal	herb and/or lemon
chocolate flavoring	seasoning
junk food snacks	fructose—available in
	powder and capsule form
	whole-grain cereal
	carob

fresh fruit, pop-corn
(unsalted, without butter)

Self-Health Foods

To help give you a better feel for this diet and also to provide you with an easy shopping and menu planning guide, here is a breakdown of priority foods you should make a point of including in your diet.

THE SELF-HEALTH PANTRY

Poultry: eat white meat only.

Meats: concentrate on lean cuts of veal, lamb, beef and pork.

Fish: whitefish or trout are good choices.

Vegetables: practically every vegetable—including potatoes (baked or boiled)—is fine.

Fresh fruits: any and all.

Grains: brown or wild rice, bran and whole-grain cereals.

Breads: choose whole-grain breads such as 100 percent rye, stone-ground whole wheat, and whole-grain crackers.

Fluids: ten glasses per day of any sugar-free liquid, including water (preferably bottled), skim milk, cranberry, orange, or tomato juice.

Finally make a conscious effort to avoid:

- Foods containing nitrates and sodium nitrites: bacon, lunch meats, and sausage.
- Specific seafoods: oysters, clams, lobsters, and shrimp. They are too high in cholesterol.
- Refined sugar and foods containing large amounts of refined sugars: candy, cake, cookies, ice cream, syrups, and soft drinks—to name a few.

- Products made from unenriched refined or white flour such as white bread and soda crackers.
- Processed, canned, and frozen foods to which salt has been added. Substitute herbs and/or lemon juice as seasonings for freshly prepared foods.

Knowing what to eat is only half a diet. You also must learn how to eat, how to mix and match your food combinations to get the most nutritional benefit out of them without boring your taste buds. And that's where the next chapter will help.

4
THE
SELF-HEALTH DIET

Although nutritionists have known for some time how you can compute your personal food energy needs on a day-by-day basis and how much energy there is in certain portions of specific foods, it is only recently they have been able to figure out how much of each kind of food you should eat for a truly balanced diet. For example, a forty-year-old man who is six feet tall requires about 2600 calories per day; but if he gets all 2600 from the wrong foods—1200 in chocolates and 1400 from eggs, to use exaggerated examples—he is going to look and feel lousy. It is important to know how to get calories *and* nutrition at the same time.

Fortunately, this information is now available in an easily understandable form. It is basically a matter of matching your age and ideal weight with the appropriate caloric need and the best food combination to satisfy that need. For example, in the hypothetical case above, the calorie breakdown chart used in this chapter with the self-health diet rules out a chocolate and egg diet and suggests instead that the daily quota of 2600 calories be made up as follows: 1248 from complex carbohydrates; 260 from simple carbohydrates; 520 calories from unsaturated fats; 260 calories from saturated fats; and 312 calories from proteins. By checking the tables for each of these food components you can then put together a tasty daily menu.

The information in this chapter will help you fulfill

two goals in your daily diet: the right balance of food components and the satisfaction of caloric needs.

As you saw in the last chapter, the self-health diet is designed to give you a daily food supply that is: 48 percent complex carbohydrates, 10 percent simple carbohydrates, 20 percent unsaturated fats, 10 percent saturated fats and 12 percent protein. In addition it will give you the proper balance of vitamins, minerals, and fiber.

One of the simpler ways to gauge your food needs is by food energy units or calories. Once you know how many calories you need you can compute how much food you can eat. Because of the seemingly endless procession of fad diets, many people think of calories in a totally negative context. It is true of course that calories put on weight if you consume too many, but they are also what keeps your body humming. If you consume too few, you may feel tired and dragged out. How many calories your body needs and consequently how many you should consume every day, depends on a number of variables: your age, height, ideal weight, and how active you are.

The first step in designing your own self-health diet is to figure out how many calories you need each day. The procedure is very simple. To help you do this, there are eight tables in this chapter. The first three help you find your daily caloric needs based on your age and build and they also help you gauge the number of calories you need from each of the main food groups. The remaining five tables give you a detailed breakdown of the choice of foods in each group and the number of calories per average (four-ounce) serving of each.

THE SELF-HEALTH DIET FORMULA

To get the self-health diet to work for you, simply follow these four steps:

1. Turn to Table 1, find your height in the left-hand column and then read across to the right until you hit the column that best describes your frame size: small, medium, or large. This will tell you what a person of your size and build should weigh ideally.

2. With your ideal weight and your age in mind, turn to Table 2 which shows Daily Caloric Needs. Find your ideal weight in the left-hand column—it should be within five pounds of that number—and read across until you get to the column that fits your age range. A man who is twenty-five years old, for example, with an ideal weight of 145, according to this chart needs about twenty-seven hundred calories per day.

3. Now that you have your body's daily caloric need, turn to Table 3, the Calorie Breakdown Chart. As you read across you will see how many calories you should consume from each of the five food groups—complex carbohydrates, simple carbohydrates, unsaturated fats, saturated fats, and proteins.

4. With your caloric breakdown for each food group in hand, look through each of the five food group tables. They give detailed listings of specific foods and the calorie content per serving. Use these to plan your meals—one whole day, not just one meal at a time. Your daily calorie totals won't always match your need number exactly, but try to get as close to the number as possible. The workings of the self-health diet depend on how accurately and honestly you keep track of your daily caloric intake.

One final note about starting the self-health diet: eat for your ideal weight. If you weigh 165 pounds, but your weight chart says you should be closer to 155 pounds, follow the calorie and food combination formula for the 155-pound level. It will take a little time, but eventually your real and ideal weight will be the same.

TABLE 1:   IDEAL WEIGHT*

Height	Small Frame	Medium Frame	Large Frame
FOR WOMEN			
5 ft. 0 in.	92– 98	96–107	104–109
5 ft. 1 in.	94–101	98–110	106–112
5 ft. 2 in.	96–104	101–113	109–118
5 ft. 3 in.	99–107	104–116	112–121
5 ft. 4 in.	102–110	107–119	115–125
5 ft. 5 in.	105–113	110–122	118–130
5 ft. 6 in.	108–116	113–126	121–135
5 ft. 7 in.	111–119	116–130	125–140
5 ft. 8 in.	114–123	120–135	129–145
5 ft. 9 in.	118–127	124–139	133–150
5 ft. 10 in.	122–131	128–143	137–155
5 ft. 11 in.	126–135	132–147	141–160
6 ft. 0 in.	130–140	136–151	145–165
FOR MEN			
5 ft. 4 in.	115–123	121–133	129–132
5 ft. 5 in.	118–126	124–136	132–137
5 ft. 6 in.	121–129	127–139	135–142
5 ft. 7 in.	124–133	130–143	138–148
5 ft. 8 in.	128–137	134–147	142–152
5 ft. 9 in.	132–141	138–152	147–155
5 ft. 10 in.	136–145	142–156	151–160
5 ft. 11 in.	140–150	146–160	155–165
6 ft. 0 in.	144–154	150–165	159–170
6 ft. 1 in.	148–158	154–170	164–175
6 ft. 2 in.	152–162	158–175	168–180
6 ft. 3 in.	156–167	162–180	173–185
6 ft. 4 in.	160–171	167–185	178–190

° These weights are based on the muscle–bone–fat ratio of the mod ·
erately active rather than the athletic individual. Therefore the ideal
weight for a very active person with excellent muscle tone may exceed
the specified weight by 3 or 4 percent.

TABLE 2: DAILY CALORIC NEEDS AT YOUR IDEAL WEIGHT

Desirable Weight	Age 18–35	Age 35–55	Age 55–75
WOMEN			
Calories			
99	1,700	1,500	1,300
110	1,850	1,650	1,400
121	2,000	1,750	1,550
128	2,100	1,900	1,600
132	2,150	1,950	1,650
143	2,300	2,050	1,800
154	2,400	2,150	1,850
165	2,550	2,300	1,950
MEN			
Calories			
110	2,200	1,950	1,650
121	2,400	2,150	1,850
132	2,550	2,300	1,950
143	2,700	2,400	2,050
154	2,900	2,600	2,200
165	3,100	2,800	2,400
176	3,250	2,950	2,500
187	3,300	3,100	2,600
198	3,550	3,250	2,700

TABLE 3: DAILY CALORIC BREAKDOWN

Total Daily Calories	Complex Carbo- hydrates Table 4	Simple Carbo- hydrates Table 5	Unsat- urated Fats Table 6	Saturated Fats Table 7	Proteins Table 8
1300	624	130	260	130	156
1400	672	140	280	140	168
1500	720	150	300	150	180
1600	768	160	320	160	192
1700	816	170	340	170	204
1800	864	180	360	180	216
1900	912	190	380	190	228
2000	960	200	400	200	240
2100	1008	210	420	210	252
2200	1056	220	440	220	264
2300	1104	230	460	230	276
2400	1152	240	480	240	288
2500	1200	250	500	250	300
2600	1248	260	520	260	312
2700	1296	270	540	270	324
2800	1344	280	560	280	336
2900	1392	290	580	290	348
3000	1440	300	600	300	360
3100	1488	310	620	310	372
3200	1536	320	640	320	384
3300	1584	330	660	330	396
3400	1632	340	680	340	408
3500	1680	350	700	350	420
3600	1728	360	720	360	432

TABLE 4: COMPLEX CARBOHYDRATES

Food (4 oz. serving unless otherwise specified)	Calories per average serving
Apples (fresh, 1 med.)	90
Apples (dried, uncooked)	320
Apple juice	57
Applesauce (canned)	45
Apricots (raw, 1 med.)	25
Apricots (dried)	445
Artichokes (1 lrg.)	50
Asparagus	23
Bananas (1 med.)	100
Beans, lima	115
Beans, string	29
Beans, red	115
Beans, pinto	265
Bean sprouts	15
Beets	38
Blackstrap molasses	60
Blueberries	57
Bran	115
Broccoli	29
Cabbage	23
Cantaloupe (½ med.)	30

Source: *Nutrition and Physical Fitness*, 8th Edition. L.J. Bogert, T.M. Briggs, D.H. Calloway. W.B. Saunders Company, Canada, 1966.

(Table 4:   continued)

Food (4 oz. serving unless otherwise specified)	Calories per average serving
Carrots	38
Cauliflower	29
Celery	20
Corn	100
Cucumber (½ med.)	7
Dates	265
Grapefruit (½ med.)	40
Grapes	265
Honey (1 tbsp.)	60
Lemons (1 med.)	29
Lemon juice (½ cup)	25
Lentils (cooked)	115
Lettuce	15
Macaroni and cheese	230
Milk	
whole (1 cup)	165
low fat (1 cup)	110
skim (1 cup)	85
Mushrooms	35
Oatmeal (¾ cup)	65
Oranges (1 med.)	75
Orange juice	55
Onions, green	5
Peaches (1 med.)	45

(Table 4:   continued)

Food (4 oz. serving unless otherwise specified)	Calories per average serving
Pears (1 med.)	110
Peas	80
Pepper, green (1 med.)	15
Pineapple	57
Potatoes	
baked (1 med.)	95
french fried (20 pieces)	275
mashed (½ cup)	95
Rice	
brown	115
white	115
Sherbet	135
Spaghetti marinara	145
Spinach	29
Squash	20
Strawberries	25
Tomatoes	25
Tomato juice	20
Vinegar, 1 tbsp.	5
Watermelon	29
Wheat germ (1 tbsp.)	35
Yeast, brewer's (1 tbsp.)	23
Yogurt, low fat	57

TABLE 5: SIMPLE CARBOHYDRATES

Food (4 oz. serving unless otherwise specified)	Calories per average serving
Beer (12 oz.)	150
Biscuits (1 med.)	108
Bread (1 slice)	60
Cake: chocolate, fudge icing (1 slice)	370
pound cake (1 slice)	125
Candy: butterscotch (1 oz.), chocolate (1 oz.), hard (1 oz.)	115
caramels (1 oz.)	120
chocolate with almonds (1 oz.)	160
marshmallows (1 oz.)	100
Cookies (3 small or 1 large)	120
Crackers, saltine (1)	17
Ice cream	250
Jams and preserves (1 tbsp.)	55
Liqueur (1 oz.)	100
Pancakes (1 med.)	50
Pie (1/6 of 9-inch pie): apple	410
blackberry	390
cherry	420
custard	350
lemon meringue	360
mince	435
pumpkin	320
Rum (1.5 oz.)	150
Sugar: brown (½ cup)	410
white, granulated (½ cup)	385
(1 tbsp.)	66
(1 tsp.)	22
powdered (1 cup)	495
(1 tbsp.)	45
(1 tsp.)	15

Waffles, from mix with milk and eggs (1)	205
Whiskey (1.5 oz.)	110
Wine: dry, 20 percent alcohol (4 oz.)	160
light dry, 12 percent alcohol (4 oz.)	100
sweet, 20 percent alcohol (4 oz.)	180

TABLE 6: UNSATURATED FATS

Food (4 oz. serving unless otherwise specified)	Calories per average serving
Almonds (1 oz.)	166
Avocados	177
Coconut (1 oz.)	100
Margarine, from vegetable oil (1 tbsp.)	100
Mayonnaise (1 tbsp.)	109
Salad oil (1 tbsp.)	125
Sunflower seeds (1 oz.)	142
Peanuts (1 oz.)	142
Peanut butter (1 oz.)	166
Walnuts (1 oz.)	200
Chocolate, bitter or baking (1 oz.)	150
Pecans (6 med.)	105
Salad dressings, commercial (1 tbsp.)	
blue cheese	80
French	60
French, low calorie	15
mayonnaise	100
thousand island	75

TABLE 7: SATURATED FATS

Food (4 oz. serving unless otherwise specified)	Calories per average serving
Bacon (1 strip)	52
Butter (1 tbsp.)	100
Corned beef	400
Frankfurters	320
Lamb	285
Pork	571
Pork sausage (1 link)	95
Bologna	320
Cheese (1 oz.)	
cheddar	120
cream	110
American cheese food (e.g. Velveeta)	95
American	85
Chile con carne: with beans (1 cup)	335
without beans (1 cup)	500
Cream (¼ cup)	
half and half	80
heavy, or whipping	210
light	130
Ham, smoked, cooked (2–3 small slices)	290
Oyster stew, 1 part oyster, 3 parts milk (1 cup)	200
Salami (1 oz.)	135
Sausage, Vienna, canned (2 oz.)	145

TABLE 8: PROTEINS

Food (4 oz. serving unless otherwise specified)	Calories per average serving
Abalone	115
Bass, striped	228
Beef, choice steak	320
Beef and vegetable stew	94
Bluefish	125
Bonito	200
Brains	142
Butterfish	114
Carp	114
Cheese: cottage (¼ cup)	60
Swiss (1 oz.)	110
Chicken	285
Clams	87
Cod	200
Crab meat (½ cup)	100
Eggs: omelet (2 small eggs)	175
white (1)	16
yolk (1)	64
Fish sticks	200
Gelatin, dry, plain (1 tbsp.)	35
Halibut	200
Ham (2 med. slices)	290
Hamburger	
regular	245
lean	185
Liver	228
Lobster, canned or cooked (⅔ cup)	95
Mackerel	285
Oysters, raw (5-8 med.)	100

Table 8: (continued)

Food (4 oz. serving unless otherwise specified)	Calories per average serving
Parsley, raw (1 tbsp.)	2
Perch	115
Pike	102
Salmon	210
Scallops: raw (3½ oz.)	80
breaded, fried (3½ oz.)	195
Shrimp	130
Soy beans (½ cup)	120
Tongue, beef (3½ oz.)	245
Tuna	150
Veal: cutlet, broiled (3½ oz.)	215
shoulder, oven braised (3½ oz.)	235

YOU AND YOUR SELF-HEALTH MENU

Maybe you were a little surprised to see some of the restricted foods listed on these tables. You shouldn't be. Just because a food is restricted doesn't mean you have to cross it off your daily menu forever. As long as that piece of chocolate cake or ice cream cone fits in your day's caloric-nutrition formula there's no reason why you can't have it. After all, this is a diet you should be able to follow for the rest of your life. And what's life without that occasional chocolate-chip cookie, piece of pie, or glass of white wine?

Of course sometimes it takes a little manipulating to get the daily diet to accomodate some of these extravagances, but if you're good with numbers you can probably use these tables to come up with satisfying dessert-day menus. One simple technique is to limit your intake of liquids to no-cal drinks such as water, plain tea, or black coffee. Maybe the following menus will give you some other ideas. They are all designed to satisfy a daily caloric need of twenty-four hundred calories. The components of each meal are labeled for their food grouping and calorie content. The following letter code is used:

CC = Complex Carbohydrates
SC = Simple Carbohydrates
UF = Unsaturated Fats
SF = Saturated Fats
P = Proteins

If you take the time to study the menus you'll see that they give you a good cross section of foods. There are no villain food components in this diet. Don't make the mistake of assuming certain types of foods are automatically bad for you. Even people who have a higher than average awareness of nutrition sometimes think wrongly that one type of food is superior to another. Of course you need protein, but you also need carbohydrates and fats. What you don't need is an excess of them. Probably nothing illustrated this more dramatically than the tragedies that came out of the liquid-protein diet fad. In 1978 there were fifty-eight people who literally dieted themselves to death by ingesting little else but very low-calorie, predigested "liquid" protein. Accept the fact that no lifelong diet can be that simpleminded (and boring) and you will have instantly immunized yourself against the lure of the latest fad diet.

Menu # 1—for 2400 Calories Total Daily Requirement

Breakfast:

	Calorie Count
3 pancakes (SC)	150
honey, 5 tbsp, (CC)	300
2 tbsp. margarine (UF)	200
orange juice (CC)	55
skim milk (CC)	85

Lunch:

fruit and nut salad

orange (CC)	75
grapefruit (CC)	40
apple (CC)	90
banana (CC)	100
walnuts–1 oz. UF)	200
½ cantaloupe (CC)	30
watermelon (CC)	30
wheat germ (CC)	35

Dinner:

baked ham (P)	290
scalloped potatoes (CC)	100
with cheese (SF)	290
vegetable salad:	
with lemon juice and pepper	29
broccoli (CC)	29
cauliflower (CC)	29
carrots (CC)	38
squash (CC)	20
½ slice blueberry pie (SC)	150
skim milk (CC)	85

Daily Calorie Total

complex carbohydrates	1141
simple carbohydrates	300
unsaturated fats	400
saturated fats	290
proteins	290
Total	2421

Menu # 2

	Calorie Count
Breakfast:	
oatmeal (CC)	65
½ cantaloupe (CC)	30
whole milk (CC)	165
Lunch:	
peanut butter sandwich:	
peanut butter (UF)	666
2 slices bread (SC)	120
honey (CC)	60
banana (CC)	100
apple-grapefruit salad (CC)	130
whole milk, 1 cup (CC)	165
Dinner:	
veal scallopine (P)	320
baked potato (CC)	95
salad:	
lettuce (CC)	15
tomato (CC)	25
carrots (CC)	38
celery (CC)	20

cucumber (CC)	7
bean sprouts (CC)	15
yogurt dressing (CC)	37
cheddar cheese (SF)	120
wine (SC)	180

Daily Calorie Total

complex carbohydrates	967
simple carbohydrates	300
unsaturated fats	666
saturated fats	120
proteins	320

Total	2373

Menu # 3

	Calorie Count
Breakfast:	
1 egg (P)	88
2 bacon (SF)	104
1 cup whole milk (CC)	165
1 biscuit (SC)	108
pineapple juice-8 oz. (CC)	114
2 tbsp. margarine (UF)	200
Lunch:	
salad	
lettuce (CC)	15
carrots (CC)	38
cucumber (CC)	7
tomato (CC)	25
potato (CC)	95
salad dressing (UF)	140
apple (CC)	90
cheese (SF)	110
apple juice-8 oz. (CC)	114

Dinner:
  chicken (P)   285
  rice (CC)   115
  salad:
    lettuce (CC)   15
    carrots (CC)   38
    cucumber (CC)   7
    tomato (CC)   25
    salad dressing (UF)   140
  pear (CC)   110
  whole milk (CC)   165

Daily Calorie Total
complex carbohydrates   1138
simple carbohydrates   108
unsaturated fats   480
saturated fats   214
proteins   373

                        Total   2313

Menu # 4

Breakfast:
  omelet:
    2 eggs (P)   170
    tomato (CC)   25
    avocado (SF)   177
    ½ cup whole milk (CC)   82
    1 tbsp. margarine (UF)   100
  whole wheat toast (SC)   60
  1 tsp. margarine (UF)   33
  orange juice (CC)   57

Lunch:
gazpacho soup:
    cucumber (CC)   7
    green pepper (CC)   15
    tomato (CC)   25
    green onion (CC)   5
    2 tsp. wine vinegar (CC)   10
    2 cups tomato juice (CC)   40
fruit salad:
    orange (CC)   75
    grapefruit (CC)   40
    pear (CC)   110
    walnuts –1 ounce (UF)   200
skim milk (CC)   85
½ roll with margarine (SC)   55

Dinner:
spaghetti marinara (CC)   145
    —with meat sauce (P)   185
salad:
    lettuce (CC)   15
    cucumber (CC)   7
    bean sprouts (CC)   15
    tomato (CC)   25
    carrots (CC)   38
    mushrooms (CC)   35
    2 oz. raisins (CC)   160
    cheddar cheese (SF)   110
    salad dressing (SC)   70
fruit cup
    banana (CC)   100
    strawberries (CC)   25
    pineapple (CC)   55
glass of red wine (SC)   100

Daily Calorie Total

complex carbohydrates	1196
simple carbohydrates	285
unsaturated fats	333
saturated fats	287
proteins	355
Total	2456

Menu # 5

	Calorie Count
Breakfast:	
fruit salad:	
orange (CC)	75
apple (CC)	90
strawberries (CC)	25
walnuts– 1 oz. (UF)	200
oatmeal (CC)	65
toast (SC)	55
margarine (UF)	100
decaffeinated coffee	0

Lunch:	
Malibu salad:	
lettuce (CC)	15
celery (CC)	20
spinach (CC)	29
red and green cabbage (CC)	23
green onions (CC)	5
broccoli (CC)	29
young green peas (CC)	80
carrots (CC)	38
mushrooms (CC)	35

bean sprouts (CC)	15
sunflower seeds (UF)	142
tomato (CC)	25
cucumber (CC)	7
sweet green pepper (CC)	15
salad dressing (UF)	70
banana (CC)	100
glass of white wine (SC)	100

Dinner:

chicken (P)	285
–braised in wine (SC)	100
rice (CC)	115
asparagus (CC)	23
–in cheese sauce (SF)	110
skim milk (CC)	85
sherbet (CC)	135
1 roll (SC)	108
margarine (UF)	100

Daily Calorie Total

complex carbohydrates	1049
simple carbohydrates	363
unsaturated fats	612
saturated fats	110
proteins	285
Total	2419

Menu # 6

Breakfast:	*Calorie Count*
bran (CC)	115
honey (CC)	60
skim milk (CC)	85
banana (CC)	100
dates (CC)	265
toast (SC)	60
margarine (UF)	100

Lunch:	
salad:	
lettuce (CC)	15
tomato (CC)	25
cucumber (CC)	7
bean sprouts (CC)	15
yogurt dressing (CC)	57
apple juice (CC)	57
fruit salad:	
strawberries (CC)	25
orange (CC)	75
apple (CC)	90
walnuts-2 oz. (UF)	400

Dinner:	
baked halibut (P)	200
fresh asparagus (CC)	23
salad:	
spinach (CC)	29
tomato (CC)	25
carrots (CC)	38

1 egg (P)	85
1 oz. parmesan cheese (SF)	110
lemon juice (CC)	25
skim milk (CC)	85
chocolate fudge cake (SC)	185

Daily Calorie Total

complex carbohydrates	1216
simple carbohydrates	245
unsaturated fats	500
saturated fats	110
protein	285
	————
Total	2356

Menu # 7

	Calorie Count
Breakfast:	
2 waffles (SC)	410
margarine (UF)	100
orange juice(CC)	55
skim milk (CC)	85
honey–2 tbsp. (CC)	120

Lunch:	
tuna salad:	
tuna (P)	150
celery (CC)	20
egg (P)	85
tomato (CC)	25
fruit salad:	
cantaloupe (CC)	30

watermelon (CC)	29
strawberries (CC)	25
wheat germ (CC)	35
walnuts (UF)	200
coconut (UF)	100
skim milk (CC)	85
sherbet (CC)	135

Dinner:
Milano minestrone soup:

onions (CC)	5
tomato paste (CC)	25
celery (CC)	20
carrots (CC)	38
zucchini (CC)	20
brown rice (CC)	115
beans (CC)	265
potatoes (CC)	95
1 pear (CC)	110
Gouda cheese–2 oz. (SF)	220
decaffeinated coffee (black)	0

Daily Calorie Total

complex carbohydrates	1227
simple carbohydrates	410
unsaturated fats	400
saturated fats	220
protein	235
Total	2492

SELF-HEALTH DIET SUPPLEMENTS

The Four Energizers

If you're looking for some safe food additives to add to your foods and give yourself a lift, try one or more of these: brewer's yeast, yogurt, blackstrap molasses, and wheat germ.

Brewer's yeast is a valuable addition to your diet because it is such a rich source of B vitamins and minerals. It is a low-calorie food, twenty-three calories per table-spoon, but it is packed with sixteen amino acids, fourteen minerals, and seventeen vitamins. You can get it at most health-food stores. If you decide to use it, take about two tablespoons of it in your diet each day.

Eaten plain or as a higher-calorie flavored snack, yogurt is a good source of high-quality protein, calcium, and vitamin B. The bacteria in it also act to aid your digestion. A four-ounce daily serving of yogurt is a good idea. That adds about fifty-seven calories to your complex carbohydrate quota.

Blackstrap molasses offers an equally broad nutri-tional plus. It contains more calcium than milk, more iron than most eggs, and more potassium than most foods. A tablespoon a day will also boost your vitamin B intake.

Finally, wheat germ is also an excellent source of protein, B-complex vitamins, vitamin E, and iron. It's available in supermarkets in wheat-germ form and in health-food stores both as wheat germ and as wheat-germ oil.

You can use the four energizers any way your taste and imagination suggest. You can sprinkle wheat germ on cereals, use the yogurt in salads, or even mix them all together. Combining brewer's yeast, blackstrap molasses, and wheat germ in a pint of yogurt will give you a tremendously nutritious food.

The Self-health Drink

As a nutritious and refreshing alternative to that calorie-laden beer or sugary soft drink, mix your own substitute: the self-health drink. The ingredients are simple and the only special equipment you need is a blender. It's so nutrition-rich, you can drink a twelve-ounce glass of it as a substitute for breakfast or lunch. Depending on your preferences you can make it with either fruit or vegetable juice.

To make a quart of the self-health drink, start with one quart of any of the following:
  orange juice
  pineapple juice
  tomato juice
  carrot juice
  celery juice
  or any other fruit or vegetable juice.

To this add:
  1 tablespoon blackstrap molasses
  1/2 cup brewer's yeast
  1 tablespoon wheat-germ oil

And if you want to experiment with flavoring the drink, try adding any or all of these ingredients:
  lemon
  honey
  fruit pulp

When everything has been put in, mix it in your blender and store it in your refrigerator. It's a vitamin-rich, tasty drink that goes well with meals.

LOSING WEIGHT THE SELF-HEALTH WAY

As I mentioned earlier, the point of the self-health diet is not primarily to lose weight. It's to get you into the life-saving habit of good nutrition. If you weigh more than you should according to the charts in the beginning of this chapter, you probably will lose some weight by following your self-health diet formula. But before you get into the specifics of how to do that, you should recognize some of the basic facts of life about dieting.

Just remember this one fact and you will have the key to any workable diet: *the only sensible way to lose weight is to reduce your calorie intake.* Period. There are no magic foods, no special pills, no fancy equipment that will lose weight for you safely and healthfully. Nutritionists say that many of the popular diets work, for a while. But they also warn that since many of these diets require either too much or too little of the food the average human body needs, healthy individuals cannot—and should not—stick to them for very long.

Experts also note that it is pointless to lose weight unless you seriously intend to maintain that lower weight. And if you are serious about getting down to a lower weight and staying there, the best thing for you to do is discuss what your best weight should be with your doctor and between the two of you work out a diet that will get you down to that and keep you there.

There are various tricks you can try to help you along:

count calories religiously; skip all snacks; use a smaller plate for smaller portions (so you don't seem to be eating less); put your fork down between bites; slow down your eating pace by chewing longer; and, of course, start an exercise program. These all will help you keep your calorie intake down and help you keep your weight where you want it.

But these are all just diet aids. Nothing will work until you start dropping some of those calories from your meals. Just by eating a hundred fewer calories each day you can lose ten pounds a year. If you want to lose a little more weight or lose it more quickly just take your customized self-health diet and cut your daily caloric allowance in half. If your caloric intake should be three thousand, drop it to fifteen hundred. This will enable you to lose up to three pounds each week.

Before you rush ahead, there are three things you should remember. First, never let your daily allowance dip below nine hundred calories. You can't possibly get enough nutrition if you do. Secondly, always observe the basic self-health formula of choosing a balance of foods from each of the five component groups following the recommendations for the size and number of servings for your calorie level. Finally, once you have mapped out your diet consult your physician before you start on it.

You have a long list of foods to choose from; if you are looking for something to snack on or as a low- or no-calorie accompaniment to a meal, always think in terms of fresh vegetables, fresh fruits, canned fruits with no sugar, plain tea or coffee, cocoa powder for flavoring, water ices, gelatin, and puddings made with nonfat milk. Be extremely frugal with frozen or canned fruits containing sugar, and with honey, jellies, jams, ice cream, fried foods, and certain high-calorie nuts such as walnuts.

An ideal diet aid, one that will help you keep your weight where you want it, is a good exercise program. A really good exercise program, of course, is much more than that. It is a rejuvenator and ultimately a lifesaver. And that's what you have in the second half of the self-health fitness program.

5
SELF-HEALTH
IN ACTION:
SHAPING
A YOUNGER BODY

Y ou probably know that exercise can help you feel better, and look better. But did you know that it can literally *make* you younger as well? One of the more surprising discoveries that has come out of research into exercise is that in addition to slowing down the aging process, it can actually reverse some of its effects. Not very many people ever bother to take advantage of this fact. In fact, most of us seem to do the least amount of exercise at a time in our lives when we need it the most.

Although it's barely perceptible, the process of aging begins while you're still in your early twenties and continues over the years. Gradually your heart loses some of its ability to pump blood. Your blood pressure rises a little (or a lot if you're not on a self-health diet). Part of the reason is arteriosclerosis, a condition in which the inner diameter of your arteries shrinks because of fats collecting in them.

Your muscles lose some of their power. You may have to strain a little more to do the same work that never bothered you when you were younger. The capacity of your lungs shrinks. One result of this is that your body's ability to perform slows down. Even your bones feel the effects of aging. You lose some body minerals and the bones become more fragile, more subject to breaks and fractures.

Other influences also take their toll. Pollutants in our environment, bad health habits, and years spent watching sports on television instead of playing them help speed the aging process. What is worse is that many of us simply give in. Usually the reason given is something like, "The damage is already done. Why worry about it? It's too late now to do anything."

That is not true. To take just one example of the rejuvenating effect of exercise, a University of Wisconsin study found that a steady regimen of workouts actually reversed the age-induced loss of minerals from the bones of one group of people. What was even more remarkable was the people for whom this worked. Their *average* age, the researchers reported, was eighty-four.

Studies such as this have shown that even after years of abuse, your body is forgiving and adaptable. It has a resilient, natural urge to stay healthy. And with the self-health exercises you can tap this urge. Based on sound research into exercise and physical fitness the self-health exercises offer a series of activities that in twelve weeks will have you feeling better than you have in years. You will look better, have a more buoyant step, actually be able to see your skin glow with good health, and enjoy the kind of endurance you haven't had since your childhood.

Even if you're one of those people who see exercise as a penance, you'll be pleasantly surprised by the self-health technique. It is not a crash exercise course, so don't expect to have to submit yourself to one of those ordeals like some of the last-ditch exercise routines you may have put yourself through a week or two before the skiing or tennis season. And it is not an endless ritual of repeating the same boring exercises over and over. Variety is automatically built into the self-health exercise program.

Adaptability is as well. Whatever kind of shape you are in, whatever your exercise needs, the program can be customized to suit you. It will work equally well for:

- *The beginner*: in just twelve weeks you will have moved through the conditioning program to better health and better appearance.
- *The moderately active*: this is a program which is easy to adapt to your present schedule for greater fitness and well-being.
- *The very fit*: those who are already in condition can look forward to a new program with more variety than any they have ever tried.

The regimen can be adapted to those with special needs: for the person on a very tight schedule, for the individual who wants to exercise indoors or outdoors, and for the traveler who wants to maintain fitness while on the road. And a special senior program has been designed for the older health-conscious person.

PHYSICAL PERFORMANCE

As you prepare yourself for any exercise or sport, it helps to have some understanding of the elements that determine the effectiveness of your performance. Knowing what these are will assure you of the best possible results from your efforts.

As you've seen, aging works on two features of your body. First, your circulation slows down. Second, you begin to lose some of the strength and endurance you had when you were younger. What self-health exercise offers is a program that will directly counteract both those effects, giving you sets of activities that will improve the power of your heart and blood circulation as well as showing you how to maintain and improve your whole body's strength.

Energy output

To get the most out of these techniques, you first have to know how to get the most out of yourself, especially, your personal energy sources. Every cell in your body is a microscopic combustion engine. To operate at peak efficiency each of these cells needs two things: fuel and oxygen. The fuel it gets from glycogen, a kind of car-bohydrate, and fatty acids. The oxygen comes from hemoglobin, the pigment in your red blood cells that carries oxygen from your lungs to other parts of your body. The more your cells work, the more fuel they burn and the more oxygen they need.

Doctors can measure how much oxygen your body needs both at work and at rest. In general, they know that for every liter of oxygen you take in, a certain amount of energy, five kilocalories, is released in your body. Most commonly they find this by putting someone on a moving treadmill or bicycle to study his or her oxygen use, or uptake. By knowing how much oxygen a person is taking in at peak performance, at top speed on the treadmill or bicycle, they can determine the maximum power of that person's energy-burning combustion engine. Since oxygen is transported by your blood, this measurement is also an indirect way of showing how big a load your heart and circulatory system can handle. The greater your oxygen uptake at full speed—technically called the maximum aer-obic, or oxygen-using, power—the greater your heart's ability to pump.

Not all exercise or heavy work depends wholly on the blood–oxygen relay system. As you first start working out, the muscles can work as an anaerobic, or oxygenless, engine. The cells manage to split up energy-rich substances such as glycogen into less energy-rich fuels, which they can burn without oxygen. The only problem is that your muscles can do this for only a very short time.

Unless the aerobic, oxygen-fueled system can take over, a kind of poison called lactic acid builds up in your muscles as a byproduct of anaerobic activity. The muscles are overwhelmed by this substance; they stiffen and refuse to obey orders. This often happens when you've pushed yourself so far past your peak-performance level that the anaerobic motor takes over.

To exercise at the peak of your efficiency for longer stretches of time you have to have a more efficient aerobic engine working. And the only way to develop it is by exercises that make your lungs work, such as swimming, bicycling, walking, and running. They stretch your power capacity. No exercise program is worth anything without these aerobics, as they're called. Your body can't be trained to use its energy efficiently without them.

Your neuromuscular training

Even with a high level of aerobic power, you are still not going to perform any sport or exercise smoothly and efficiently without your nervous system, the wiring of your body, operating at its best. All bodily movement involves a complicated interplay between different groups of muscles. This coordination isn't possible without your central nervous system. The system works somewhat like a computer. Your spinal cord is the trunk line of this computer. Contained in it are the nerve cells which extend their fibers to the muscle cells in the body's trunk and its extremities.

Impulses generated in these nerve cells activate the muscle cells via the nerve fibers. Every move you make involves these nerve cells. They exert a tremendously complex control system that activates some muscle groups while inhibiting others, all to give you a specific movement.

Some of these movements are automatic, but most are things your body learns as you grow and develop. This means that as you become proficient at doing something—walking as a child, to use a very basic example—a certain wiring pattern in your nervous system is set up. You have a distinct pattern of sequential nerve-cell actions that let you put one foot in front of the other, use all the proper leg muscles to move you along and keep you perfectly balanced, and keep a certain muscle rhythm going to make the motion fluent.

Our senses feed into this computer system telling us when we're doing things wrong and when we've got it right. This kind of feedback improves that special feature of performance called technique, which is the ease and efficiency with which we perform an exercise or movement. Having the physical strength and endurance to do a certain exercise is never enough. You have to take the time to get your nervous system in shape as well. Practicing a certain movement does more than flex your muscles and skeletal system, it tunes up your nervous system as well, making it much more efficient at that movement. The effect of this is to make your body more efficient at using its energy as well as exercising a less visible part of your body, those nerve cells that keep it functioning smoothly.

Psychological factors

Even more elusive and intangible is that certain state of mind that lets you benefit from your exercise. If you've done any exercising on a regular basis or played a sport before, you know that sometimes you're in the mood for it and sometimes you're not. Often there's no particular reason for this. Physically you may feel perfectly fine, but mentally you may be indifferent or feeling drained. This psychological attitude has a tremendous influence on your performance.

Your mind is a powerful and often underestimated component in exercise. You probably know, for example, that even on your down days you can will your body into action with some mental effort, but researchers have also found that under unusual situations, such as in hypnosis or moments of extreme danger, or even where you're getting a tremendous jolt of encouragement—the cheering crowd at the finish line—you may suddenly find that your mind has got your body performing beyond what you thought its limits were. Just knowing that this mind power is there should help you get through some of your sluggish exercise days.

Of course, you can't have a cheering crowd gather around every time you have a bad day. But there are some tricks to help yourself adjust. You can switch over to different exercises to alleviate the boredom or slacken up on the pace a little or even adapt other tactics such as the one used by people with respiratory conditions or cardiac problems. Even with these difficulties a person can do heavy work if he or she absolutely has to by taking frequent micro-pauses, ten- to thirty-second rest breaks alternating with ten- to thirty-second spells of work. Don't think you have to be exercising at white-hot intensity all the time to benefit. Doing any exercise, no matter how slowly, is always better than doing none at all, if you do it regularly.

Be aware of the fact that all these factors—your body's energy efficiency, how well rehearsed it is, even your state of mind—can affect your ability to perform. By being aware of them and adjusting your regimen accordingly, you can get the most from your workout on any given day.

Finally, your personality has a lot to do with how you exercise. Not everyone is all that interested in physical exercise. At one extreme are those who believe that if men and women were meant to exercise, they would be born with lifetime memberships in a health spa. These skeptics see any activity that makes a person perspire and breathe hard as a peculiar way to pass the time. At the other extreme are the physical-fitness fanatics who sleep with their running shoes on and are obsessed with their mileage, running times, and marathons. If you're like most people, you probably fall somewhere between these two extremes. You realize exercise is important, but just can't seem to stick with an exercise program. Or if you exercise now, you're not sure if you're doing the right workouts or if you're doing them enough. Maybe even somewhere in the back of your mind is lurking the doubt that it's going to do you any good at all.

Exercise and the new you

At this point, it might help to review exactly what a habit of exercise can do for you. As I mentioned at the beginning of this chapter, one decided benefit is to slow down and reverse some of the wear and tear of the aging process. "So many people rust out before they wear out," observes one exercise expert, appropriately named Dr. Robert E. Wear, of the University of New Hampshire. He and other experts have found that a habit of exercise is about the closest thing we have to a fountain of youth.

Even if you consider yourself in good health now—no particular ailments to worry about—you can improve through exercise. For example, take two fifty-year-olds identical in physical endowment, but different in another aspect. One has a habit of exercise that's been kept reasonably well through life, while the other spends most spare time in front of the TV set. Put on a treadmill or bicycle, the exerciser would most likely show an oxygen-uptake ability from 20 to 30 percent higher than the TV watcher. In other words, the exerciser would have the physical condition of the average person ten to fifteen years younger.

Exercise increases your capacity to do physical work. By working the muscle tissue, it slows down the loss of that tissue which routinely comes with aging. Research by German doctors has shown that exercise even improves your nervous system. The more you use your nerve cells, it seems, the longer they last. Doctors have found that exercise is especially good for your joints. Older people who routinely exercise have fewer arthritic problems in their hips than people of the same age who lead sedentary lives. By whittling away at the known risk factors, exercise may well lengthen your life.

Obesity

Just a hundred extra calories in your daily diet will produce ten extra pounds on your body in just one year. To weigh less you must eat fewer calories. As you may already know this is not the hard part of dieting, at least not in the beginning. The hard part is, once you've arrived at your ideal weight, to stay there. And this is where exercise can help.

Don't fall into the trap of believing in an exercise-and-eat-anything-you-want diet. Exercise does help you burn up calories but it may not be as efficient at it as you think. For example, to lose one pound you have to burn up thirty-five hundred calories. Now if you decide to go out and jog away this extra pound, you would have to run a little over thirty miles. Exercise is primarily for fitness, for muscle tone, for boosting your body's strength and endurance.

But it can be an excellent companion for a good diet because it does help you keep your weight down where you want it. Although it can't, and isn't meant to, take the place of a diet, it can make it much easier to follow one since it does act as kind of a safety valve in letting you eat and enjoy more calories than you could as a strictly sedentary person.

In this way it helps you avoid the health risks of being overweight: the added stress on your circulatory and respiratory systems, the threat inherent in high blood pressure and cholesterol buildup, and the danger of diabetes and heart disease.

Heart disease and stroke

Helping to keep your weight down isn't the only way exercise puts more distance between you and heart problems. It keeps the muscles of your heart in shape. Hearts fail because they become weak. They simply can't pump the volume of blood to your lungs and the rest of your body that they once could. Failed hearts are muscles that have lost their strength and their endurance.

Many times this happens simply because that muscle hasn't been flexed enough. It is not all that difficult to do. There are many circulatory-respiratory exercises that work the heart and lungs, build up the strength and endurance of the whole body system. It is now a well-known medical fact that regular circulatory-respiratory exercises lessen the chance of a heart attack and, even if one does occur, lessens its severity.

The exercises improve general circulation, increase the oxygen-carrying abilities of the blood, reduce blood cholesterol, expand blood supplies to the heart muscle, and in general help the heart to do the same amount of work with much less effort. Even after heart attacks these exercises speed a victim's recovery.

The President's Council on Physical Fitness, after reviewing the enormous amount of research on the subject, reached these same conclusions. It found that done long enough, hard enough, and steadily enough, exercises such as bicycling, swimming, and jogging could all produce these salutary effects on your body.

Exercise and your mind

The longer you continue with your exercise habits the greater will be your natural vigor and sense of vitality. The reason is quite simply that the machinery of your body is better tuned. Besides the physical benefits, there are certain mental pluses. Being fit improves your attitude about yourself. Things you once had difficulty doing—sports, exercises, daily chores—will come easier to you. The increase of muscle strength and endurance will enable you to enjoy your leisure time with family and friends that much more.

This was confirmed in a complex research project known as the Medford, Oregon Boys' Growth Study in which one group of boys was studied for eleven years, from their seventh to their eighteenth birthdays. Researchers found a positive relationship between physical fitness and personality characteristics. The boys who scored high on physical motor tests were more outgoing, more active, and more likely to be popular. Those who scored low tended to feel inadequate, insecure, and socially ill at ease. They were more likely to be defensive and rebellious.

Similar profiles have resulted from groups of adults measured before and after going through a self-health exercise regimen. As they got into the exercise program, the adults became more adventurous, more emotionally stable, more composed and relaxed in their life outlook. Conversely, physical deterioration causes social and psychological deterioration as well. It doesn't take much thinking to see how feeling good physically translates into feeling good mentally. The ease and power that comes to your body from regular exercise can have a infectiously uplifting influence on your whole outlook.

And there are still more benefits. In a report entitled *The Brain, Too, Has Arteries*, the cardiologist Dr. Paul Dudley White pointed out that keeping a good circulation of blood flowing to the brain is tremendously important for developing and maintaining intellectual well-being. The quality of this circulation depends on the strength of your heart, the strength of your diaphragm, and the blood-pushing capacity of your leg muscles. All these muscles are important because the heart is not a vacuum pump. When your body is upright, the heart cannot draw the blood up from your feet and legs all by itself. When you move your legs, when your leg muscles contract and pulsate, you help your heart work against gravity and circulate the blood throughout the body and to the brain in particular.

Studies of both children and adults have found that learning potential increases with physical fitness. After twenty-four years of studying intellectually gifted children, Stanford psychologist Dr. Lewis M. Teman says that the popular image of the child genius as being undersized, sickly, and nervous couldn't be further from the truth. He has found that the gifted child is likely to be more physically fit than the average. Although this high level of fitness hardly accounts for the child's level of intellect it is obviously an important contributing factor.

Stress

If you already exercise occasionally, you may also be aware of another special benefit of exercise: a safety valve for stress. That special feeling runners and athletes talk about at peak performance can at least partially be explained by special things that happen biochemically.

Among its other effects, exercise releases two important neurotransmitters, norepinephrine and serotonin, into the bloodstream. These chemicals are manufactured by the brain to control pain and depression, as well as to transmit nerve impulses throughout the brain. These chemicals are especially important during times of stress. On these occasions your body reacts by releasing adrenaline, levels of which are also determined by how much you exercise. Adrenaline is a precursor to serotonin and norepinephrine, which act as natural chemical buffers to protect you against the impact of stress. Studies have shown that individuals deficient in these chemicals tend to feel tired and listless. They are also more vulnerable to the depression that comes with severe stress. In short, stress cuts into your supply of these two chemicals and the less of them you have, the more brutal will be the impact of stress on your system.

Studies have also shown that you can raise your serotonin and norepinephrine level and keep it high by exercise. By increasing your production of neurotransmitters, you simultaneously increase your natural protection against stress and the depression that sometimes comes with it.

THE FIVE PRINCIPLES OF EXERCISE

As you can see, there is a lot to gain by the self-health exercise habit: a more energetic and supple body; a heart that beats stronger and steadier; a physique with better coordination, balance, and endurance; a more self-confident you; a zest for life; and automatic insurance against the general effects of aging as well as against specific risk factors that reduce your life span.

As you get ready to start your self-health exercise program and to enjoy its benefits, you should understand and apply the five principles of exercise. Let these shape your attitude and planning and you will be able to get the most out of the program. They are simple, common-sense notions, but like so many simple things, they are sometimes overlooked.

1. Tolerance

Your body has its own special needs as well as its own strengths and weaknesses. As you start the exercise program, you will get a clearer sense of what they are. Be attuned to your body. The self-health program is flexible enough to suit just about every normal exercise need. Don't be afraid to experiment or vary what you do until you get the right combination. This will help you find your limits in different areas. And once you know these, you can get a clearer sense of how to slowly guide your body past those limits to higher levels of fitness. You will also be able to set up your personal programs so that you can fully exercise your body without exhausting it.

2. Assessment

Many people believe they have reached their exercise tolerance before they really have. Quite often this limit is a purely psychological one. For that reason you should stop now and again to take a good look at just how you are progressing. As a beginner you should raise your tolerance level gradually over the first two months. By the end of that time regular exercise will be as much a part of your day as eating and sleeping. This is when some tend to get complacent about their exercise. In the long run, this complacence tends to deprive you of benefits you could be getting by trying to stretch yourself a little at a time. This is where your periodic assessment helps. If you are completely honest with yourself, you'll be able to tell when you are working up to your exercise potential and when you are just coasting. Exercise helps your body come alive and stimulates a natural appetite for more exercise. Don't coast, feed this appetite. It will do you a world of good.

3. Overload

The name for this stretching technique is a misnomer in a way. The idea of any good exercise program is to take yourself slightly beyond your present exercise tolerance. At first it will seem like overloading but if it is done right, you'll be amazed at how easily and smoothly your body responds to the challenge. The benefits from this are increased circulatory-respiratory fitness, greater strength, and an extension of endurance. Once you have gauged your tolerance correctly and can periodically assess it with an experienced eye, the overload technique will become a part of your exercise habit.

4. Progression

Once you get in the habit of finding your tolerance, assessing your new level, and building in that careful overload of exercise, progress will follow naturally. Your strength and stamina will grow. Think in terms of moving forward by increasing the amount of time and intensity with which you exercise. This kind of program will involve your mind as much as your body.

5. Commitment

Finally, none of these principles will be worth anything without your making a solid commitment to good health. To be physically fit and stay that way, you must make exercise a part of your life. This may call for some adjustment in your thinking. You can't be a weekend athlete and expect to get any substantial physical benefit. If anything, you're probably taking too many risks by occasionally overtaxing an unprepared body. For your continued good health you need a steady routine of exercise as much as you need food and water. Once you've come to believe in it as a necessity for a good life and act on your belief, you've already taken a giant step in the direction of total self-health.

6
THE
SELF-HEALTH
EXERCISE
PROGRAM

If you're willing to take just twelve weeks of your time to grow a little younger, the self-health exercise program is for you. In three months' time or even sooner, depending on your present physical condition, you can look forward to a longer life, an overall glow of good health, and a more youthful appearance.

This regimen assumes you are moderately active but not in the habit of daily all-round vigorous physical exercise. For example, if you play golf or tennis a couple of times a week, those games may help some of your muscles, but they do not give you a totally conditioned body. In fact, no leisure-time sport provides for balanced development of all parts of the body. The self-health exercise plan does.

The program is a graduated series of exercises especially chosen to develop your circulatory and respiratory system as well as improve your strength and endurance. There are two types of exercise, one for each of these goals, as well as a series of warmup exercises you should do at the beginning of each session. The exercises are grouped so that they can be done in carefully planned clusters five times a week.

There are three stages. Depending on your physical health, you may start in the first or skip ahead to the third. Wherever you begin, you will have a plan to increase your level of tolerance. Chances are that after several weeks of workouts, you will find it hard to believe how far and how fast you have advanced. As your physical tolerance for exercise increases, so will your psychological tolerance. The program provides its own initiative, giving you a trimmer appearance, a growing energy for daily work, more zest for play, and a general feeling of well-being that will keep you hooked on fitness.

As you get ready, there are a few things to remember to help you progress more smoothly. The most important thing to note, if you remember nothing else, is to take it easy. Don't try to rush the program, to do too much too soon. When you begin you will probably find that some of the exercises make you a little sore. If you pace yourself properly, the soreness will disappear in a short time. By starting slowly and carefully, you avoid the sudden strains and minor injuries that delay progress. There is no hurry, so don't push yourself, especially during the first eight weeks of the program. You are building a lifetime habit of exercise here and projects like this do take a little time.

You can avoid many problems simply by practicing the five principles of exercise. Listen to your body. It will signal you when you are moving too quickly. If, after an exercise session, you have headaches, nagging back pain, nausea, insomnia, or a crippling stiffness and soreness the next morning, you are overdoing it. During the initial adjustment period your body will need some time to get used to this new regimen. You may find you need more sleep or that, during one of the sessions, you can't do as long a series of exercise repetitions as the program suggests. Obey your better instincts: stop during the exercises for a short breathing spell and continue only when you feel stronger—and get to bed earlier. You'll be surprised to see how soon those aches disappear, how soundly you'll sleep, and how easily you'll be able to run through those exercises that once gave you trouble.

WHEN TO EXERCISE

You are the best judge of what is the "right" time to exercise. For early risers, the so-called larks of the world, the morning is when they have all their pep and vigor and when they are most inclined to do their workouts. For the late people, the "owls," a better time could be late afternoon or early evening. You may have to experiment a little, but eventually you'll find the hour or so that suits you. While you're thinking of possible times, don't forget your lunch hour. Working out then is a good way of avoiding a high-calorie lunch and becoming healthy at the same time. The important thing is not what time of day you exercise, but doing it faithfully five days a week up to an hour a day.

WHERE TO EXERCISE

Depending on the type of workout you choose, you can do it in a swimming pool, on a local athletic field, in your backyard, or even in your living room. Most likely on pleasant days when it's still light out, you'll want to be outdoors. At those times the easiest place to work out is probably your local high-school athletic field. If you live near a big park or an open stretch of land, so much the better. But you don't need a great deal of room to follow the program.

WHAT TO WEAR

Wear whatever is comfortable. It can be anything from an old T-shirt and shorts to a monogrammed warmup suit. A good rule of thumb is to wear natural fibers, such as cotton and wool. In the summer cotton absorbs perspiration and helps keep you cool and in the winter woolen mittens, ski cap, and sweater will keep you warm even when you are damp with perspiration. That old exercise standby, the plain gray cotton sweat shirt, is perfect. You don't need fancy clothing. And you certainly don't need gimmicks like rubber exercise suits. Those can be dangerous, especially on warm days. They trap body heat and can expose you to the risk of heat stroke.

On your feet a good pair of cotton or woolen (if it's cold) socks will do fine, along with a pair of comfortable sneakers. If you plan to include jogging in your exercise program, invest in a good pair of running shoes. These are specially designed to help protect your feet and legs from the brutal punishment they take during a run. (Sneakers are not built to do this and will do you more harm than good.) They're your best insurance against sore, blistered feet and aching knees and ankles. Nylon shoes are a good bet because they are light and will stay soft even after being soaked by rain or wet grass.

FIGHTING THE BIG B: BOREDOM

You hear it all the time: "I used to exercise, but it was so boring I stopped." Maybe that's an excuse or maybe it isn't, but many people do throw over their exercise plans for that reason. If you give it a little thought, you can avoid this trap. One of the best methods is to do some of your workouts with a friend. Even if it's only a couple of times a week, it will help you to have someone with you.

It also helps to ingrain exercise into your daily life so that it becomes an automatic and necessary part of your day. The simplest way to do this is to schedule your sessions for the same time each day.

If you exercise indoors, you might be able to distract yourself on days when your motivation is not the highest. Listening to your favorite records or radio program while exercising might help the time pass more quickly. Or you can take some of the guilt out of watching TV by scheduling your exercise times to coincide with your favorite shows or a big game you can't miss.

The self-health program is adaptable and has a built-in insurance against dullness. You can vary the exercises and still follow it. You can customize the program to your own life style and preferences. Often what appears boring is no more than an exercise you are not comfortable with. Keep experimenting until you get what you want.

Lastly, to keep your interest up and to fine-tune your awareness of how well you are doing, take the time to chart your progress. You'll find a sample chart at the end of each stage. Seeing the evidence of your progress on paper can give you the psychological lift you need on those tough days.

BEFORE YOU BEGIN: CAUTION

Check with your doctor before you start the self-health exercise regimen, particularly if:

- you have not had a physical examination within the last year
- you are over thirty and your life style has been sedentary
- you are overweight or have a history of high blood pressure or heart disease.

Under these circumstances or if you have any doubts or questions at all, show this program to your doctor. If you are perfectly healthy, he or she will probably give you unconditional support and approve your good sense. Even if you have a medical problem that stands in the way of your full participation in the program, you and your doctor may be able to work out a modified version to suit your particular needs.

GIVE YOURSELF A FITNESS TEST

The first part of the self-health program tests your state of physical fitness and helps you determine your exercise tolerance level. With this test you will be able to judge just where you should start, in which of the three stages. The test was adapted from tests developed by the President's Council on Physical Fitness.

1. Walk Test

You have ten minutes for this. How many minutes can you walk on a level surface at a fast pace without difficulty and discomfort?

- If you have to stop and rest before having walked for five minutes, start the self-health exercises at Stage I (p. 131).
- If you can walk for more than five minutes but have to stop and rest before completing ten minutes, begin the program at the third week of Stage I (p. 132).
- If you can walk for the full ten minutes, but you find yourself tired and winded at the end, begin the program at Stage II (p. 135).
- If you can easily walk for the full ten minutes at a good fast pace without a break, then take the walk-jog test.

2. Walk–Jog Test

Alternately walk fifty steps and jog fifty for ten minutes.

- If you have to stop and rest before the ten minutes are up, begin the exercise program at the third week of Stage II (p. 137).
- If you can complete the ten minutes, but find yourself tired and winded at the end, begin the program at the last week of Stage II, then move on to Stage III (p. 140).
- If this ten-minute test was hardly a challenge to you, begin the program at Stage III.

Now that you have tested your level of fitness, you're ready to start the self-health program. Turn to the stage that suits you and begin. Use your common sense. Don't push yourself too hard. Listen to your body. If you can do more than is required in the early part of the stage, move on to a more challenging level. Ultimately your body will decide how much exercise is right for you.

The number of exercises vary from one stage to the next but what remains the same is the structure of each stage. Each uses three types of exercises: warmups, circulatory-respiratory exercises (or C-R for short), and conditioning exercises designated by the code S-E, for strength and endurance.

You *must* spend the first five minutes of every exercise session doing the warmups. These loosen up your muscles and joints, increase circulation and respiration, and help build up your body heat to stretch muscles and connective tissue and prevent injuries. Always do these for five minutes.

Circulatory-respiratory, or C-R, exercises are designed to increase the fitness of your heart, blood vessels, and respiratory system. You will have a choice of these as well as conditioning, or S-E, exercises designed to flex each of the major muscle groups. The variety of choice enables you to switch the elements of the program and keep it interesting and challenging.

HOW TO APPLY THE PROGRAM

Each daily series involves eight exercise sets. Half of these are C-R exercises; half are S-E exercises. So as not to wear you out, the exercises are alternated, and the strength and endurance exercises, as you will notice, are set up with a certain pattern in mind. First they exercise your shoulders, then the arm and chest area. Then they flex your abdomen and waist muscles, lower back and buttocks, and finally give your feet and legs a workout. As you work on your regimen, experiment with the different types, and when you find the ones you like best, write them down.

All the exercises are described in the next few pages. Most of them you probably already know. The self-health plan is not based on exotic postures or fancy equipment. The secret of its effectiveness is in ordering the exercises in a special sequence. Read through the description of the exercises first, and once you have a sense of how they are done, turn to the exercise program on p. 131.

WARMUP

No matter what your stage or level of fitness, you must warm up for five minutes before exercising. The warmup exercises will stretch your muscles, ligaments, and tendons; raise your body temperature; and get your circulatory and respiratory systems tuned up and ready to work. The warmup will make exercising more comfortable and prevent injuries.

1. Stretch and bend

Stand with feet about shoulder width apart. Extend hands straight up and reach as high as possible and hold this position for five to six seconds. Bend from the waist, flexing knees slightly. Gently stretch and try to touch toes. Hold for about thirty seconds, breathing deeply. Repeat two to three times.

2. Knee pull

Lie on back with hands at sides. Bend left leg up to chest, hold with both arms for about five seconds, stretching gently. Repeat with the other leg. Stretch each leg seven to ten times.

3. Arm circles

Stand erect, arms straight out at shoulder height, palms up. Move arms in small backward circle fifteen times. Reverse direction and move arms in small forward circles. Do this fifteen times.

4. Body bender

Stand with feet about shoulder width apart, hands interlaced behind head. Bend sideways from waist to the left as far as possible. Repeat to the right. Bend ten times each side.

If you have access to a swimming pool and choose in-the-water exercise for your C-R and S-E exercises, you can use any of the warmup exercises above. If you do not choose the C-R and S-E water exercises, but wish only to warm up in the water, try these:

5. Side bender

Stand in waist-deep water with right arm down at side and left arm extended overhead. Stretch slowly and bend to the right. Return to starting position. Repeat. Reverse: left arm at side and right arm overhead. Warm up with this exercise for about thirty seconds.

6. Stride hop

Stand in waist-deep water with hands on hips. Jump, pushing left leg forward and right leg back. Jump again, bring right leg forward and left leg back simultaneously. Repeat for about fifteen seconds.

CIRCULATORY-RESPIRATORY (C-R) EXERCISES

These are expressly designed to develop your heart, lungs, and circulatory system. The best way to monitor yourself as you do the exercises is to check your heart rate or pulse. To derive the greatest benefit, the exercises should be done at 70 to 80 percent of your maximum heart rate. As you get older, the maximum heart rate declines, so what applies for you today is not true ten years from today. The simplest way to find out your ideal exercise pulse is to consult the following table:

If you are at or close to (5 years) the age of:	70% of your maximum heart rate is:	80% of it is:
20	140	155
30	135	150
40	130	145
50	125	140
60	120	135
70	115	130

Divide your maximum heart rate by six. This is the

number of times your heart should beat in ten seconds during the peak of your exercise activity. To find out if you are working at the proper intensity, exercise for a while then stop. Now take your pulse either from your wrist or the carotid artery, which is in your neck. Take it for a count of ten seconds, multiply by six and compare the resultant figure to the figure from the chart.

You should get in the habit of routinely checking your pulse rate during exercise sessions and adjust your exercise so that you are within a few beats of your target rate. Ideally you should be able to work yourself up to your target rate for thirty minutes or more a day, four or five times each week without feeling too fatigued. With this kind of simple pulse guide you should be able to tell if you are trying to go too far too fast or not fast enough.

The following are the C-R exercises you will be able to use:

1. Jumping rope

An excellent aerobic exercise, jumping rope can be done indoors as well as outdoors at whatever pace suits your current conditioning. It does wonders for your coordination and upper body development as well as your cardiopulmonary system. You can either skip with both feet off the ground or with alternating feet using a kind of running in place motion.

2. Jogging

There's little to know about technique for this sport except to run with your back straight, head up, and arms slightly away from your body, forearms parallel to the ground. To minimize the shock to your legs and feet run on soft earth or on a gravel track if you can, not concrete or asphalt. Make sure to wear running shoes, not sneakers, for this.

Relax, breathe deeply as you run, with your mouth open. Take short steps, landing on your heel and rocking forward, driving off the ball of your foot. If for any reason you become unusually fatigued or uncomfortable, slow down, walk, or stop. Jog with your heart beating at 70 percent of your maximum heart rate for the time specified. Walk for thirty seconds before and after each C-R exercise.

3. Walking

Walking is often the forgotten exercise. For too many of us our cars have taken the place of our legs. Now is the time to get them back into shape. Consider making walking a permanent part of your exercise routine. It can take the place of running and it offers certain advantages. It is not as hard on your body. You are less likely to suffer the kinds of foot, leg, and knee injuries that plague runners. Walking can give you just as much muscle tone and, as an added bonus, you see more as you walk. For this reason it is more than an exercise, it's an experience. Move your walking tempo up to a brisk pace, going uphill if you feel fit enough, to get your 70 percent maximum rate.

4. Bicycling

Bicycling is an excellent toning exercise for your upper as well as lower body and it offers great circulatory-respiratory benefits. Since it can be a nuisance climbing off a regular bike to do your other S-E exercises, you might want to include bicycling when you are indoors and there is a stationary exercise bike available. As with the other exercises, pedal at your 70 percent level for the exercise time specified and give yourself a thirty-second cooldown of slow pedaling or walking before and afterward.

5. Swimming

Use any type of stroke you favor for this exercise and swim for the specified time at your 70 percent maximum giving yourself a thirty-second slow swim before and after each exercise set.

6. Interval swimming

Again you can use any kind of stroke. Here you will swim for a specific distance. Once you've done that, swim slowly back to your starting point or get out of the pool and walk back. This will be your cooldown exercise.

7. Bobbing

1. Stand in shallow water.
2. Take a deep breath.
3. With feet touching the pool bottom, submerge your body in a tuck position, and exhale while submerged.
4. Shove off bottom and stand again.
5. Inhale. Repeat this for the specified number of times, and bob with your heart working at 70 percent of maximum.

STRENGTH AND ENDURANCE (S-E) EXERCISES

Each one of these is designed to build up specific areas of your body, mostly by repetitive exercise sets. There are two general kinds: those you can do in your living room, back yard, or recreation field; and those you can do in a pool. First, the dry land exercises:

1. Ankle stretch

Stand on a large book or a block of wood with your weight on the balls of your feet and heels hanging over the edge of the book. Raise heels slowly, then lower them. Repeat.

2. Arm circles

Stand erect, arms straight out from your sides at shoulder height with palms up. Move arms in small backward circles for the specified number of repetitions. Now reverse direction and move arms in small forward circles for the same number of repetitions.

3. Back leg raiser

Lie on your back. Raise legs to vertical position. Now slowly lower them to the ground. Repeat.

4. Chin-up

Standard: grasp the chin-up bar with both hands, palms forward. Lift your body off ground till your chin clears the bar. Lower body slowly, all the way down to the starting position and repeat.
Alternate: stand at arms length facing a wall. Place your hands against the wall. Lean in to the wall and push away. Repeat specified number of times.

5. Flutter kick

Lie face down with hands under your thighs. Arch your back to bring the chest and head up. Now flutter kick your legs from the hips with knees slightly bent.

6. Half knee bend

Stand erect with hands on hips. Extend arms forward and simultaneously squat halfway. Return to starting position and repeat.

7. Hop

Standing erect, hop on both feet at once for the specified number of repetitions.

8. Knee push-up

Lie face down with legs together and knees bent, feet raised off the floor. Place hands on the floor, palms down, shoulder width apart. Push upper body off the floor until arms are fully extended. Return to starting position. Do specified number of repetitions.

9. Leg thrust

Sitting, with both hands on floor behind you to support your weight, tuck both knees toward chest, then thrust legs out straight. Repeat specified number of times.

10. Midsection raise

With your back toward floor, supporting body on hands and heels (reverse of push-up position), whip midsection of body up and down rapidly. Repeat specified number of times.

11. Prone arch

Lie face down, hands under thighs. Raise head, shoulders, and legs from floor. Return to starting position. Repeat specified number of times.

12. Prone arch, hands extended

Same as prone arch, except arms are extended to either side at shoulder level.

13. Push-ups

Lie on the floor with legs together and hands on the floor about shoulder width apart. Now push your body off the floor so that your weight is supported on your hands and toes. Then slowly lower your body until chest touches the floor. Keep the body straight at all times during this exercise.

14. Right-left hop

Hop on your right foot for the specified number of times and then switch to your left foot for hopping the same number of times.

15. Side leg raise (slow)

Lie on your right side, right arm extended straight out, supporting head. Your left arm should be in front of your chest with the palm of your hand on the floor. Slowly lift your left leg about two feet off the floor. Slowly lower it and repeat this specified number of times. Now roll over and repeat on the other side.

16. Side leg raise (rapid)

Lying on your right side, right arm supporting your head, whip left leg up and down rapidly, lifting it as high as you can off the floor. When you've done the specified number of repetitions, repeat this on your other side.

17. Side leg raise (on extended arm)

Lying on right side, support your rigid body with right foot and right extended arm. Hold left arm behind head and raise left leg as high as you can. Then lower it. After doing the specified number of repetitions, roll over and repeat on your other side.

18. Sit-ups (arms extended)

Lie on your back with legs together and arms extended above head. Bring arms up and over head and roll up to a sitting position. Slide hands along the top of your legs. Grasp ankles. Now roll back to the starting position and repeat.

19. Sit-ups (fingers laced)

Lie on back with legs straight out in front of you, fingers laced behind head. Curl up to a sitting position and touch left elbow to right knee. Lie down again. Curl back up to a sitting position. This time touch right elbow to left knee. Return to starting position. Score one sit-up for each time you return to starting position.

20. Sit-ups (fingers laced, knees bent)

This is the same as sit-ups (fingers laced) except that you lie on your back, knees bent, feet flat on floor. Do sit-ups as before.

21. Sprinter

Squat like a frog with hands on floor. Extend left leg to the rear. Quickly reverse the position of your feet in a bouncing movement. Switch your feet again and return to starting position.

22. Toe-ups

Face the wall at arm's length. Lean forward, with hands on the wall. Raise yourself up and down on toes.

23. Wide arm circles

Stand erect with feet shoulder width apart, hands hanging loosely at your sides. Raise arms out to each side, bring them up and forward and cross them over head while still moving. This should complete a full circle in front of your body. Do equal sets of these first with arms rotating forward, then in the opposite direction.

24. Wing stretcher

Stand erect with elbows raised to shoulder height, fists

clenched in front of chest. Quickly thrust elbows back, but do not arch your back. Return to starting position and repeat.

STRENGTH-ENDURANCE (S-E) WATER EXERCISES

If you are a swimmer you can stay in the pool and continue your self-health exercises for strength and endurance. As you will notice, all of these are to be done in the shallow end of the pool in water that is anywhere from waist to chest deep.

25. Alternate toe touch

As you stand in the water, raise left leg. Then, twisting right shoulder forward, try to touch left foot with right hand. As you do this look back over left shoulder slightly while extending left hand to the rear. Return to your standing position and do the same thing with right leg and left arm. Repeat specified number of times.

26. Knees-up twister

With your back toward the side of the pool, hold on to the gutter with both arms fully extended behind you to each side. Draw knees up to chest. Twist slowly to the right. Return to starting position. Twist slowly to the left. Return to starting position. Repeat for the specified length of time at a moderate pace.

27. Leg out

Stand at the side of the pool with your back against the wall. Raise left knee to chest, extend the leg straight out, and stretch it. Drop the leg to starting position. Repeat. Then reverse to other leg. Repeat for the specified length of time at a moderate pace.

28. Raising hips

Facing the side of pool, hold on to the pool gutter with one hand and put the other hand flat on wall so you can push legs out. Raise hips and hold for four counts. Now relax. Repeat this cycle.

29. Side bender

Stand in waist-deep water with right arm at side and left arm straight overhead. Stretch, slowly bending to the right. Return to starting position. Repeat. Now switch to left arm at side and right arm overhead. Repeat for the specified length of time at a moderate pace.

30. Standing crawl

Stand in waist- to chest-deep water. While standing, simulate the overhand crawl stroke: reach out with the left hand, press downward and pull the left hand through to the thigh. Repeat this with your right hand. Repeat for the specified length of time at a moderate pace.

31. Toe bounce

Stand in waist- to chest-deep water with hands on your hips. Jump high, keeping feet together. Repeat for the specified length of time at a moderate pace.

32. Walking twist

Stand in waist- to chest-deep water. With fingers laced behind head, lift right leg and twist body so you can touch your right knee with your left elbow. Drop your leg and now do the same thing with your left leg and right elbow. Repeat for the specified length of time.

STAGE I

Do these exercises once a day, five days a week. They are marked C-R and S-E so that you can see what they are designed to do: C-R are circulatory-respiratory exercises, S-E are muscle strength and endurance exercises, and "reps" means repetitions.

WEEK 1

Since this will be your first week, pace yourself carefully. If at any time during this week you become out of breath, simply slow down or stop until you get it back.

Special note: always do your five minutes of warmup exercises before each exercise session.

Warmup—five minutes

    1. C-R: do one of the following:

        walk: briskly, 2.5 minutes
        swim: 1 minute
        bicycle: briskly, 2.5 minutes
        bob: 2 times, 10 reps. each time
        jump rope: 2.5 minutes, 50 times per minute

    2. S-E: do one of the following:

        knee push-ups: 6 reps.
        arm circles: 20 reps. each way
        wing stretcher: 20 reps.
        standing crawl: 15 seconds

    3. C-R: do one of the following:

        walk: briskly, 2.5 minutes
        swim: 1 minute
        bicycle: briskly, 2.5 minutes
        bob: 2 times, 10 reps. each time
        jump rope: 2.5 minutes, 50 times per minute

WEEK 2

Do the same exercises as you did in Week 1 but this time do them at a slightly faster pace. Make sure you don't go faster than you feel you need to.

WEEK 3

The durations and times of the exercises will pick up a little here so you may feel a bit strained at first. Take your time and go at a rate that is comfortable for you.
Warmup—5 minutes

1. C-R: do one of the following:

   walk: briskly, 4 minutes
   swim: 1.5 minutes
   bicycle: briskly, 4 minutes
   bob: 3 times, 10 reps. each time
   jump rope: 60 turns a minute for 2 minutes

2. S-E: do one of the following:

   push-ups: 4 reps.
   wide arm circles: 10 reps.
   standing crawl: 30 seconds

3. C-R: do one of the following:

   walk: briskly, 4 minutes
   swim: 1.5 minutes
   bicycle: briskly, 4 minutes
   bob: 3 times, 10 reps. each time
   jump rope: 60 turns a minute for 2 minutes

4. S-E: do one of the following:

sit-ups (arms extended): 15 reps.
side leg raise: 12 reps. each leg
side bender: 30 seconds

5. C-R: do one of the following:

walk: briskly, 4 minutes
swim: 1.5 minutes
bicycle: briskly, 4 minutes
bob: 3 times, 10 reps. each time
jump rope: 60 turns a minute for 2 minutes

6. S-E: do one of the following:

prone arch: 12 reps.
flutter kick: 30 reps.
knees-up twister: 30 seconds

7. C-R: do one of the following:

walk: briskly, 4 minutes
swim: 1.5 minutes
bicycle: briskly, 4 minutes
bob: 3 times, 10 reps. each time
jump rope: 60 turns a minute for 2 minutes

8. S-E: do one of the following:

toe-ups: 10 reps.
ankle stretch: 17 reps.
toe bounce: 30 seconds

WEEK 4

This is almost the same as Week 3. This set of exercises should be done at a slightly faster pace. Also increase your S-E exercise by two or three repetitions (whichever is comfortable) or by fifteen seconds, if they are duration exercises. When you have completed the fourth week of the self-health exercises, you are finished with Stage I and are now ready to move on to Week 1 of self-health exercises Stage II.

Sample progress chart

STAGE I

Week	1	2	3	4
WARMUP FOR 5 MINUTES				
Exercises 1. C–R				
2. S–E				
3. C–R				
4. S–E				
5. C–R				
6. S–E				
7. C–R				
8. S–E				

STAGE II

All the basic rules of exercises apply here as well. Do these once a day five times a week and always precede each exercise session with a five-minute warmup.

WEEK 1

Warmup—5 minutes
1. C-R: do one of the following:

   walk: briskly, 5 minutes
   swim: 1.75 minutes
   bicycle: 5 minutes
   bob: 4 times, 10 reps. each time
   jump rope: 70 turns a minute for 2 minutes

2. S-E: do one of the following:

   push-ups: 7 reps.
   wide arm circles: 15 reps.
   standing crawl: 1 minute

3. C-R: do one of the following:

   walk: briskly, 5 minutes
   swim: 1.75 minutes
   bicycle: 5 minutes
   bob: 4 times, 10 reps. each time
   jump rope: 70 turns a minute for 2 minutes

4. S-E: do one of the following:

   sit-ups (arms extended): 20 reps.
   side leg raise: 15 reps each leg
   side bender: 1 minute

5. C-R: do one of the following:

   walk: briskly, 5 minutes
   swim: 1.75 minutes
   bicycle: 5 minutes
   bob: 4 times, 10 reps. each time
   jump rope: 70 turns a minute for 2 minutes

6. S-E: do one of the following:

   sprinter: 16 reps.
   flutter kick: 35 reps.
   alternate toe touch: 1 minute

7. C-R: do one of the following:

   walk: briskly, 5 minutes
   swim: 1.75 minutes
   bicycle: 5 minutes
   bob: 4 times, 10 reps. each time
   jump rope: 70 turns a minute for 2 minutes

8. S-E: do one of the following:

   toe-ups: 15 reps.
   ankle stretch: 20 reps.
   toe bounce: 1 minute

WEEK 2

Do the same exercises as in Week 1, but increase the pace.
Increase S-E exercises by 4 reps. or 15 seconds, the jump
rope to 75 turns.

WEEK 3

Warmup—5 minutes

1. C-R: do one of the following:

   walk 1 minute, jog 20 seconds, walk 1 minute,
       jog 20 seconds, walk 1 minute
   swim: 2 minutes
   bicycle: briskly, 20 seconds, slowly, 1 minute
       (repeat 3 times)
   bob: 5 times, 10 reps. each time
   jump rope: 80 turns a minute for 2 minutes

2. S-E: do one of the following:

   push-ups: 12 reps.
   chin-ups: 5 reps.
   standing crawl: 1.5 minutes

3. C-R: do one of the following:

   walk 1 minute, jog 20 seconds, walk 1 minute,
       jog 20 seconds, walk 1 minute
   swim: 2 minutes
   bicycle: briskly, 20 seconds; slowly, 1 minute
       (repeat 3 times)
   bob: 5 times, 10 reps. each time
   jump rope: 80 turns a minute for 2 minutes

4. S-E: do one of the following:

   sit-ups: (fingers laced): 20 reps.
   leg thrust: 20 reps.
   side bender: 1.5 minutes

5. C-R: do one of the following:

   walk 1 minute, jog 20 seconds, walk 1 minute,
      jog 20 seconds, walk 1 minute
   swim: 2 minutes
   bicycle: briskly, 20 seconds; slowly, 1 minute
      (repeat 3 times)
   bob: 5 times, 10 reps. each time
   jump rope: 80 turns a minute for 2 minutes

6. S-E: do one of the following:

   flutter kick: 40 reps.
   prone arch: 15 reps.
   alternate toe touch: 1.5 minutes

7. C-R: do one of the following:

   walk 1 minute, jog 20 seconds, walk 1 minute,
      jog 20 seconds, walk 1 minute
   swim: 2 minutes
   bicycle: briskly, 20 seconds; slowly, 1 minute
      (repeat 3 times)
   bob: 5 times, 10 reps. each time
   jump rope: 80 turns a minute for 2 minutes

8. S-E: do one of the following:

   toe-ups: 20 reps.
   hop: 20 reps.
   toe bounce: 1.5 minutes

WEEK 4

Proceed the same as in Week 3, except increase the C-R exercises to jog 30 seconds. Walk 1 minute (repeat 3 times), or swim 2 minutes at a brisk pace, or bicycle briskly 30 seconds, slowly 1 minute (repeat 3 times). Also, increase S-E exercises 2 to 5 reps. or 15 seconds, and increase your rope jumping by 10 turns, to 90 per minute for 2 minutes. When you have completed Week 4 of Stage II, you are ready to move on to Stage III.

Sample progress chart

STAGE II

Week	1	2	3	4
WARMUP FOR 5 MINUTES				
Exercises 1. C–R				
2. S–E				
3. C–R				
4. S–E				
5. C–R				
6. S–E				
7. C–R				
8. S–E				

STAGE III

The only thing that changes here is the amount of exercise. The same rules about preexercise warmups and performing the exercises five times a week still apply.

WEEK 1

Warmup—5 minutes
  1. C-R: do one of the following:

> walk 1 minute, jog 40 seconds, walk 1 minute,
>   jog 40 seconds, walk 1 minute
> swim: 3 minutes
> bicycle: briskly, 40 seconds; slowly, 1 minute
>   (repeat 2 times)
> bob: 6 times, 10 reps. each time
> jump rope: 100 turns a minute for 2 minutes

  2. S-E: do one of the following:

> push-ups: 18 reps.
> chin-ups: 9 reps.
> standing crawl: 2 minutes

  3. C-R: do one of the following:

> walk 1 minute, jog 40 seconds, walk 1 minute,
>   jog 40 seconds, walk 1 minute
> swim: 3 minutes
> bicycle: briskly, 40 seconds; slowly, 1 minute,
>   (repeat 2 times)
> bob: 6 times, 10 reps. each time
> jump rope: 100 turns a minute for 2 minutes

140

4. S-E: do one of the following:

   sit-ups (fingers laced): 30 reps.
   side leg raise: 20 reps. each leg
   leg thrust: 25 reps.

5. C-R: do one of the following:

   walk 1 minute, jog 40 seconds, walk 1 minute,
       jog 40 seconds, walk 1 minute
   swim: 3 minutes
   bicycle: briskly, 40 seconds; slowly, 1 minute
       (repeat 2 times)
   bob: 6 times, 10 reps. each time
   jump rope: 100 turns a minute for 2 minutes

6. S-E: do one of the following:

   prone arch (hands extended): 15 reps.
   flutter kick: 15 reps.
   midsection raise: 15 reps.
   raising hips: 2 minutes

7. C-R: do one of the following:

   walk 1 minute, jog 40 seconds, walk 1 minute,
       jog 40 seconds, walk 1 minute
   swim: 3 minutes
   bicycle: briskly, 40 seconds; slowly, 1 minute
       (repeat 2 times)
   bob: 6 times, 10 reps. each time
   jump rope: 100 turns a minute for 2 minutes

8. S-E: do one of the following:

   hop: 30 reps.
   toe-ups: 30 reps.
   ankle stretch: 30 reps.
   leg out: 2 minutes

WEEK 2

Warmup—5 minutes

1. C-R: do one of the following:

   walk 1 minute, jog 1 minute, walk 1 minute,
      jog 1 minute, walk 1 minute
   swim: 3.5 minutes
   bicycle: briskly, 1 minute, slowly, 1 minute
      (repeat 2 times)
   bob: 7 times, 10 reps. each time
   jump rope: 110 turns a minute for 2 minutes

2. S-E: do one of the following:

   push-ups: 20 reps.
   chin-ups: 11 reps.
   standing crawl: 2.25 minutes

3. C-R: do one of the following:

   walk 1 minute, jog 1 minute, walk 1 minute,
      jog 1 minute, walk 1 minute
   swim: 3.5 minutes
   bicycle: briskly, 1 minute; slowly, 1 minute
      (repeat 2 times)
   bob: 7 times, 10 reps. each time
   jump rope: 110 turns a minute for 2 minutes

4. S-E: do one of the following:

   sit-ups (fingers laced, knees bent): 30 reps.
   side leg raise: 25 reps.
   leg thrust: 30 reps.
   walking twist: 2.25 minutes

5. C-R: do one of the following:

   walk 1 minute, jog 1 minute, walk 1 minute
       jog 1 minute, walk 1 minute
   swim: 3.5 minutes
   bicycle: briskly, 1 minute; slowly, 1 minute
       (repeat 2 times)
   bob: 7 times, 10 reps. each time
   jump rope: 110 turns a minute for 2 minutes

6. S-E: do one of the following:

   prone arch (arms extended): 18 reps.
   midsection raise: 18 reps.
   flutter kick: 50 reps.
   raising hips: 2.25 minutes

7. C-R: do one of the following:

   walk 1 minute, jog 1 minute, walk 1 minute,
       jog 1 minute, walk 1 minute
   swim: 3.5 minutes
   bicycle: briskly, 1 minute; slowly, 1 minute
       (repeat 2 times)
   bob: 7 times, 10 reps. each time
   jump rope: 110 turns a minute for 2 minutes

8. S-E: do one of the following:

hop: 35 reps.
right-left hop: 20 reps. each foot
leg out: 2.25 minutes

WEEK 3

Proceed the same as in Week 2, but increase exercise time
and repetition. Increase the C-R set to either jog 3 minutes,
walk 1 minute (just once per set); or swim 4 minutes; or
bicycle briskly 3 minutes, slowly 1 minute; or bob 12 times.
Increase the S-E exercises by 2 to 5 reps., or 15 seconds; but
your jump-rope tempo should stay at 110.

WEEK 4

Warmup—5 minutes
1. C-R: do one of the following:

walk 1 minute, jog 4 minutes, walk 1 minute,
jog 4 minutes, walk 1 minute
interval swim: 25 yards, 5 times
bicycle: briskly, 4 minutes; slowly, 1 minute
bob: 18 times, 10 reps. each time
jump rope: 115 turns a minute for 2 minutes

2. S-E: do one of the following:

push-ups: 25 reps.
chin-ups: 15 reps.
standing crawl: 2.5 minutes

3. C-R: do one of the following:

walk 1 minute, jog 4 minutes, walk 1 minute,
jog 4 minutes, walk 1 minute
interval swim: 25 yards, 5 times
bicycle: briskly, 4 minutes; slowly, 1 minute
bob: 18 times, 10 reps. each time
jump rope: 115 turns a minute for 2 minutes

4. S-E: do one of the following:

sit-ups (fingers laced, knees bent): 33 reps.
side leg raises (rapid): 25 reps.
back leg raiser: 20 reps.
side leg raiser (on extended arm): 15 reps. each side
walking twist: 2.5 minutes

5. C-R: do one of the following:

walk 1 minute, jog 4 minutes, walk 1 minute,
jog 4 minutes, walk 1 minute
interval swim: 25 yards, 5 times
bicycle: briskly, 4 minutes; slowly, 1 minute
bob: 18 times, 10 reps. each time
jump rope: 115 turns a minute for 2 minutes

6. S-E: do one of the following:

prone arch (arms extended): 20 reps.
midsection raise: 20 reps.
flutter kick: 52 reps.
raise hips: 2.5 minutes

7. C-R: do one of the following:

walk 1 minute, jog 4 minutes, walk 1 minute,

jog 4 minutes, walk 1 minute
interval swim: 25 yards, 5 times
bicycle: briskly, 4 minutes; slowly, 1 minute
bob: 18 times, 10 reps. each time
jump rope: 115 turns a minute for 2 minutes

8. S-E: do one of the following:
hop: 38 reps.
right-left hop: 22 reps. each foot
ankle stretch: 35 reps
leg out: 2.5 minutes

Week 5

Do the same exercises as Week 4, but increase the C-R interval as follows:

jump rope: stay at 115 for 3 minutes
walk 1 minute, jog 4.5 minutes, walk 1 minute,
jog 4.5 minutes, walk 1 minute
interval swim: 25 yards, 6 times
bicycle: briskly, 4.5 minutes; slowly, 1 minute
bob: 20 times, 10 reps. each time

Also increase the S-E exercises by 2 to 5 reps. or 15 seconds.

Week 6

Do the same exercises as Week 5, and increase C-R exercises as follows:

walk 1 minute, jog 5 minutes, walk 1 minute,
jog 5 minutes, walk 1 minute
interval swim: 25 yards, 7 times
bicycle: briskly, 5 minutes; slowly, 1 minute
bob: 22 times, 10 reps. each time
jump rope: 115 turns for 3 minutes

Also increase the S-E exercises by 2 to 5 reps. or 15 seconds.

Week 7

Do the same exercises as in Week 6 and increase the C-R exercises as follows:

walk 1 minute, jog 5.5 minutes, walk 1 minute,
jog 5.5 minutes, walk 1 minute
interval swim: 50 yards, 3 times
bicycle: briskly, 5.5 minutes; slowly, 1 minute
bob: 25 times, 10 reps. each time
jump rope: 120 turns for 2 minutes

Also increase the S-E exercises by 2 to 5 reps. or 15 seconds.

Week 8

Do the same exercises as you did in Week 7 and increase the C-R exercises as follows:

walk 1 minute, jog 6 minutes, walk 1 minute, jog 6
minutes; walk 1 minute
interval swim: 50 yards, 4 times
bicycle: briskly, 6 minutes; slowly, 1 minute
bob: 30 times, 10 reps. each time
jump rope: stay at 120 turns for 2 minutes

Also increase the S-E exercises by 2 to 5 reps. and about 15 seconds.

STAGE IV AND V AND BEYOND

Once you have completed the eighth week of self-health exercise plan Stage III, you have exercised your body long enough and hard enough to be getting all the benefits of exercise described earlier. Congratulations. You are now on your way to a lifetime habit of self-health fitness. If you feel you want to increase your workouts even more, simply follow a gradual buildup. Use your common sense in pacing yourself and follow the five principles of exercise. You can't go wrong.

Sample progress chart

STAGE III

Week

	1	2	3	4	5	6	7	8

WARMUP FOR 5 MINUTES

Exercises
1. C–R

2. S–E

3. C–R

4. S–E

5. C–R

6. S–E

7. C–R

8. S–E

7
THE
EXERCISE
ALTERNATIVE

Even when you truly believe in the value of a daily exercise regimen, it is not always possible to live by that belief. For many people the obstacle might be time: one hour a day for five days a week is more than they can spare. For many, traveling in the course of work makes it difficult to find the time and space. Many older people may find five intense exercise sessions a week more than they can manage.

But even if you belong to any of these groups, you don't have to feel left out. There are three alternatives that will give you the benefits of exercise without the twelve-week self-health course. Each one is custom-designed to satisfy a specific body need.

ROVING

The first program, called roving, is for those who don't have the time to follow a full-fledged self-health program. The program is a carefully planned combination of walking and running exercises that offer you many of the benefits of the regular self-health program.

Roving will increase your body strength, stamina, and flexibility. You will feel less fatigued after a hard day's work and have more vigor and energy to spare for leisure activities with your family. Like the self-health program, it will help build a new you.

The beauty of the roving series is that it is not a long, overly complicated routine. It exercises all your muscle groups and its tempo can be adapted to your health, your own degree of fitness, and your age. You should never have trouble finding either the time or the place to perform it.

The main difference between this series and the regular self-health regimen is that you should do this one six times a week. Fortunately this is not an ironclad rule. If it doesn't fit your schedule, you can be flexible. For example, any time you feel you need a rest day, take it. If you don't like jogging or simply don't want to do it, you can substitute a brisk walk or a spell of jumping rope instead.

You should try to maintain some kind of regular schedule whatever you decide. Just to give you some encouragement, doctors who have used this alternative regimen have found that a person actually needs to do less to retain good physical shape than to acquire it.

As you will soon see, there is a pattern to the daily exercises. To help develop your body and also give it time to rest a little, exercise sessions alternate in long-short durations from one day to the next. Every week of roving exercises will follow this pattern:

Monday—short-duration exercises
Tuesday—long-duration
Wednesday—short

Thursday—long
Friday—short
Saturday—long
Sunday—rest

The roving program also follows a twelve-week format. Where you start depends on your present conditioning. To find out, give yourself the fitness test on page 117. If you are a beginner, start with Week 1. If it turns out you're moderately active, start at Week 5. If you're advanced, start with Week 9.

Week 1

Take your time as you begin. These exercises are supposed to help you, not cause you aches and pains. Start slowly to give your muscles time to warm up and ease into your pace. Since the exercises involve some jogging, it might be wise to invest in a good pair of jogging shoes. Aside from that, you need no special equipment other than a watch. One last note: if at any time you get out of breath, stop or slow down.

Day 1, 3, and 5: walk 15 minutes. Vary your pace as you go and try not to stop.
Day 2, 4, and 6: walk 5 minutes, jog 1 minute, walk 5 minutes, jog 1 minute, walk 5 minutes.
Total time: 17 minutes
Day 7: rest.

Week 2
Day 1, 3, 5: walk 15 minutes, jog 1 minute.
Day 2, 4, 6: walk 5 minutes, jog 3 minutes, walk 5 minutes, jog 3 minutes, walk 5 minutes.

Total time: 21 minutes
Day 7: rest.

Week 3
Day 1, 3, 5: walk 15 minutes, jog 1, minute.
Day 2, 4, 6: walk 6 minutes, jog 4 minutes, walk
6 minutes, jog 4 minutes, walk 6 minutes.
Total time: 26 minutes
Day 7: rest.

Week 4
Day 1, 3, 5: walk 15 minutes, jog 2 minutes.
Day 2, 4, 6: walk 3 minutes, jog 2 minutes,
repeat 5 more times.
Total time: thirty minutes
Day 7: rest.

Week 5
Day 1, 3, 5: walk 15 minutes, jog 2, minutes.
Day 2, 4, 6: walk 5 minutes, jog 5 minutes, repeat
3 times and end with a 5-minute walk.
Total time: 35 minutes
Day 7: rest.

Week 6
Day 1: walk for 30 minutes.
Day 2, 4, 6: walk 4 minutes, jog 6 minutes, repeat 2
more, ending with a 5 minute walk.
Total time: 35 minutes
Day 3, 5: walk 5 minutes, jog 10 minutes, walk 5
minutes.
Day 7: rest.

Week 7
Day 1: walk for 35 minutes.

Day 2, 4, 6: walk 4 minutes, jog 2 minutes, repeat 5
    times ending with a 5 minute walk.
Total time: 35 minutes
Day 3, 5: walk 5 minutes, jog 12 minutes, walk 5
    minutes.
Day 7: rest.

Week 8
Day 1: walk for 30 minutes.
Day 2, 4, 6: walk 2 minutes, jog 1, minute, repeat
    9 times, ending with a 5 minute walk.
Total time: 32 minutes
Day 3, 5: walk 5 minutes, jog 15 minutes, walk 5
    minutes.
Day 7: rest.

Week 9
Day 1: walk for 30 minutes.
Day 2, 4, 6: walk 1 minute, jog 30 seconds, repeat
    20 times, ending with a 5 minute walk.
Total time: 35 minutes.
Day 3, 5: walk 5 minutes, jog 20 minutes, walk 5
    minutes.
Day 7: rest.

Week 10
Day 1: walk for 45 minutes, or follow the Day three
    regimen.
Day 3, 5: walk 5 minutes, jog 20 minutes,
    walk 5 minutes.
Day 2, 4, 6: walk 15 minutes.
Day 7: rest.

Week 11
> Day 1, 3, 5: walk 5 minutes, jog 25 minutes, walk 5 minutes.
> Day 2, 4, 6: take a 15 minute walk.
> Day 7: rest.

Week 12
> Day 1, 3, 5: walk 5 minutes, jog 30 minutes, walk 5 minutes.
> Day 2, 4, 6: 15 minute walk.
> Day 7 rest.

CONTINUING

Once you have accomplished the goals of the first twelve weeks, you should level off at this plateau for four weeks. You should now be able to exercise, week in and week out without excessive fatigue or injury. After one more month of successful jogging for a certain distance, you may find you want to increase your distance.

Always increase *distance* instead of speed. In other words, it is better to travel farther at a slower pace rather than a shorter distance at a faster pace. A good rule of thumb to follow is to increase your distance by no more than 10 percent of a mile a week. After making any increase, stay at this new level for at least two to four weeks.

SELF-HEALTH FOR THE TRAVELER

All of the following exercises are weatherproof and travel-proof. You can do them anywhere you have enough room to swing your arms without hitting the walls. For those times when the weather won't let you go outside to do your regular self-health exercises, when you are just too rushed, or when you find the only place you can work out on a trip is your hotel room, do the following eleven exercises. As with all the other regimens, pace yourself according to your conditioning and always do the five-minute warmup (p.119).

1. Stretch

Stretch arms up and above your head, and then extend them out to each side slowly. Use your legs and trunk as well to make it as total a body stretch as possible.

2. Back exercise—on four counts

Clasp hands behind your back. Drop upper body forward over bent knees (count 1-2). Slowly uncurl up to standing position (count 3-4) and pull shoulders back as you finish.

3. Body twist—on four counts

This is a total-body movement using all your joints. Swing both arms sideward and upward like the blades of a helicopter, bouncing back gently for 3 counts (1-2-3). Swing arms over to other side in relaxed (knees bent) position on the count of 4.

4. Leg exercise—on four counts

Start with your feet well apart. Bend knees and try to touch palms to floor between legs (count 1). Slap hands on knees (count 2). Straighten up and clap hands together overhead (count 3). Slap hands on bent knees again (count 4).

5. Lunge—on four counts

To tone calf and thigh.
Lunge forward with left leg, knee bent, and right leg held straight behind (count 1-2-3). Jump up on the count of 4, to bring the feet together. Repeat, alternating legs.

6. Circulation

Alternating feet, roll up onto toes in a pedaling motion for 6 counts. Jog in place lifting knees high for 6 counts. Pedal again for 6 counts. Then hop forward, with your feet together, to crouch position (count 1-2). Hop back, feet together, to standing (count 3). Repeat the forward hop to crouch (1-2) and hop back to standing (count 3). Now repeat entire sequence.

7. Abdominal strength—on four counts

Lie on your back, knees bent and feet flat on the floor. Lift head, shoulders, and upper trunk, and stretch hands to knees (count 1-2). Slowly uncurl, keeping head forward, back to starting position (count 3-4). Squeeze your abdominal muscles through counts 1-2-3, and relax on 4.

8. Back and buttocks—on four counts

Start on all fours with your hands and knees on the floor. Now rock back to sit on your heels, touching chin to your knees and keeping arms outstretched on floor (count 1-2), hands still in place. Rise to original position (3-4). Now arch back and lift head while stretching one leg out and up high to the back (count 1-2). Return to original position (3-4) and repeat the cycle, stretching the other leg.

9. Cardiorespiratory: Twist-hop—on four counts

Hop twice on right foot, while pulling left knee up high and across body to touch right elbow (count 1-2). Repeat: 2 hops on left foot, etc. (count 3-4). Do at least 10 repetitions.

10. Cardiorespiratory: Leg kick

Hop on right foot, swinging left leg up in front. Hop on both feet. Hop again on left foot, swinging right leg up. Hop again on both feet. To increase the difficulty of the kick, lift leg higher and clap hands under knee on each kick. Do at least 10 repetitions.

11. Ski exercise

Hop on the spot with feet together, twisting hips so that your knees are turned to the right on count 1, to left on count 2, to right on count 3, and so forth. Relax and bend the knees with each hop. Keep arms bent and parallel to the ground, as in skiing. Do at least 10 repetitions.

EXERCISES FOR SENIORS

Age is no barrier to self-health exercises. People of every age can and should keep their bodies active every day of their lives. As an alternative to the roving exercises, an older person who wants something less taxing can try this regimen. The basic pace is whatever your ordinary walking speed happens to be. Faster speeds are whatever you can do without becoming breathless. Start out slowly to give your muscles time to limber up. Try to get in the habit of doing the exercises four or five times each week. And above all, enjoy your walk. Think of it as a planned stroll that also happens to be exercise.

1. For your warmup do:

5 minutes walking.

2. Then 5 minutes of spurt training:

Take 20-30 strides at a rapid pace, preferably uphill.
Pause for 1 minute or walk slowly for 2 to recover.
Take 20-30 strides. Recover.

Continue this for 5 minutes.

3. Now do 15-20 minutes of interval training:

Brisk walk for 2-4 minute periods.
Rest 1 minute or do slow walking between periods.

When you have improved your physical condition, so that you feel stronger and not out of breath or tired, you can add:

4. Slow jogging for 50 yards and walking for another 50.

Do this once per session. The time involved will range from 25 minutes for the totally untrained to 45 minutes when a higher level of fitness is achieved.

And remember:

- Get in the habit of exercising regularly five times a week if you can.
- Don't strain yourself. Exercise at a moderate pace, especially in the beginning.
- Vary your exercise patterns or routes to keep it interesting.
- Never exercise when you have an infection.
- Enjoy yourself. Self-health is as much a state of mind as of body.

APPENDIX:
A WALK THROUGH
THE CHEMICAL
MINEFIELD

Americans often assume we are among the healthiest people in the world. We make this assumption because we have confused technology with health. We eat abundantly but poorly. The basic facts of American life bear this out. We have added only two years to our life spans since the nineteenth century and in many areas of health we have lost ground. Heart disease, virtually unknown less than a century ago, is now the major cause of death of men over fifty. Nearly half the population suffers from some chronic illness.

As I've already mentioned, a lopsided diet and sedentary habits have done their part to contribute to this health problem, but in the past few years researchers have also found another health threat: food additives. Barely a month goes by without another additive falling under suspicion as carcinogenic or dangerous in some other way. One result of this concern about additives is a safer, if still heavily chemically saturated, diet. Unfortunately another result is panic and confusion. The attitude of "I won't eat anything I can't pronounce" has become the dietary rule of thumb for many people.

As admirable as that may be, it's not very practical. Almost every day you ingest one or another kind of food additive. The real problem is not avoiding additives but knowing which are good, which bad, and which just plain useless. Many additives are necessary as food preservatives and even may be helpful nutritionally.

This guide will help you sort out the additives to avoid. Arranged in alphabetical order are the most commonly used chemicals in our foods. Get in the habit of reading the labels on the foods you buy, especially the ones you eat most frequently. When you come across one of those polysyllabic additives, look it up here. When you do, you will be able to shop more selectively and more nutritiously as well.

As a quick reference guide, each entry is accompanied by a letter and sign code that tells you the health and safety status of each chemical—as follows:

S   = Safe for human consumption.

?   = Questionable, not fully tested or investigated.

X   = Has been shown to be hazardous. Avoid when you can.

fd   = Primarily a food chemical.

env. = Primarily a chemical you'll encounter in the environment.

ADIPIC ACID
S

This substance is sometimes added to powdered products such as gelatin desserts and fruit-flavored drinks to give them tartness. It may also be added to foods containing oils to prevent spoiling. It is not harmful to humans.

fd

ALGINATE, PROPYLENE GLYCOL ALGINATE
S

Alginate, a derivative of seaweed, is used as a thickening agent to maintain the desired texture of products such as ice cream, cheese, candy, yogurt, and canned frosting. Propylene glycol alginate is a thickening agent used to thicken acidic foods such as soft drinks and salad dressings and to stabilize the foam in beer. Both have been found to be safe.

fd

ALPHA TOCOPHEROL (VITAMIN E)
S

Vitamin E is found naturally in many foods such as whole wheat and vegetable oils. Vitamin E is added to foods to keep oils from spoiling.

fd

AMMONIATED GLYCYRRHIZIN
?

This is one of the principal flavor components of licorice. It is also used in root beer, candy, and baked goods. Ammoniated glycyrrhizin is a potent drug. Eating several ounces of licorice each day for an extended period of time has been known to cause heart failure in sensitive persons. Its relationship, if any, to cancer and birth defects has not been tested. To be safe, avoid eating excessive amounts of licorice or other candy with this ingredient.

fd

ARABINOGALACTAN (LARCH GUM)
?

This additive is used to thicken foods artificially. Short-term feeding studies on rats and dogs have not revealed any toxic effects, but lifetime feeding tests must be done before it can be considered safe for human consumption. Avoid foods containing this additive until it is fully tested.

fd

ARTIFICIAL FLAVORING
?

If you look at the list of ingredients on the label of a food package, you will see that "artificial flavoring" is frequently listed. But you are never told just exactly what ingredients make up that artificial flavoring. Food manufacturers are allowed to do this by law because as a general rule, artificial flavorings are used only in very small amounts. However, using a small amount of a chemical does not make it safe. And in the majority of cases, chemicals used for artificial flavorings have been poorly, if at all, tested for safety. Assume they are hazardous to your health until they are specifically listed on food labels and are tested and found to be safe.

fd

ASCORBIC ACID (VITAMIN C)
S

Vitamin C is added to foods such as cereals, soft drinks, and cured meats to prevent the loss of color and flavor. It is also added as an extra nutrient. It is perfectly safe.

fd

ASCORBYL PALMITATE
S

Ascorbyl palmitate is added to foods as a fat-soluble antioxidant to prevent oil-containing foods from becoming rancid. Several studies indicate that this additive is perfectly safe.

fd

AZODICARBONAMIDE
S

Used by the baking industry as a dough-conditioning agent to produce a more manageable dough and lighter loaves of bread, this additive appears to be quite safe.

fd

BENZOYL PEROXIDE
S

Benzoyl peroxide has been widely used as a flour-bleaching agent by the baking industry since 1917. Lifetime feeding experiments conducted on rats indicate that it has no adverse effects.

fd

BETA CAROTENE
S

Beta carotene is added to foods both as an artificial color and as a nutrient. It is found in such products as margarine, shortening, and nondairy creamers. The body converts beta carotene into a valuable nutrient, vitamin A. It is a safe food additive.

fd

BHA (BUTYLATED HYDROXYANISOLE)
X

BHA is an antioxidant used to retard spoilage in oil-containing foods. It has not been adequately tested for safety by long-term animal studies and therefore should be avoided.

fd

BHT (BUTYLATED HYDROXYTOLULENE)
X

BHT, like BHA, is an antioxidant commonly found in oil-containing foods such as cereals, chewing gums, potato chips, and salad oils. It is used to help products retain their freshness. BHT has been inadequately tested and therefore should be avoided until its safety has been clearly established. It has been known to cause occasional allergic reactions. Also BHT is unnecessary in many of the foods in which it is used since safer antioxidants are available.

fd

BROMINATED VEGETABLE OIL (BVO)
?

BVO is added to foods as an emulsifier and a clouding agent. It keeps oils in suspension and gives a cloudy appearance to such products as citrus-flavored soft drinks. BVO has not been adequately tested. It should be avoided. Safer substitutes are available..

fd

CAFFEINE
?

Caffeine is a mild central nervous system stimulant. It is found in coffee, tea, cocoa, and some soft drinks. It stimulates the brain, heart, and kidneys, allows one to think more clearly and to work faster, and reduces feelings of fatigue. People who drink large amounts of caffeine-containing beverages sometimes suffer from insomnia, mild fever, and irritability. Recent evidence suggests that caffeine may cause birth defects and miscarriages. As a reasonable precaution women in their first three months of pregnancy should greatly reduce their intake of caffeine-containing products.

fd

CALCIUM PROPIONATE, SODIUM PROPIONATE
S

These chemicals are added to foods such as breads, rolls, cakes, and pies to prevent the growth of mold and bacteria. They have been found to be two of the safest food additives.

fd

CALCIUM STEAROYL LACTYLATE, SODIUM STEAROYL LACTYLATE
S

These two chemicals are added to bread dough to strengthen it so it can stand up to the mechanical punishment it receives in modern bread-making machinery and also to give the bread a more uniform grain and greater volume. They also serve as whipping agents in processed egg whites and artificial whipped cream. They are easily broken down by the body and have been found safe.

fd

CARBON TETRACHLORIDE
X

Measurable quantities of this toxic chemical have been found in our drinking water. The chemical has been implicated in the two leading causes of death in the United States, cancer and cardiovascular disease. Carbon tetrachloride in our water is thought to be the result of chlorination of drinking water. As a result of chlorination, organic material in water reacts with chlorine to form this toxic chemical.

env

CARRAGEEN
S

This seaweed derivative is added to foods as a thickening and stabilizing agent. It is used to add body to soft drinks, to thicken ice cream, jelly, sour cream, and syrup and to prevent the separation of oil and water in various other products. It has been found harmless.

fd

CASEIN, SODIUM CASEINATE
S

Casein, a natural protein found in milk, is added to ice cream, ice milk, sherbet, and coffee creamers as a thickening and whitening agent. It is safe for human consumption.

fd

CHEWING GUM BASE
?

Chewing gum base is the wad that is left in your mouth when the flavor is gone from your chewing gum. It is composed of natural or synthetic chewing substances, softeners, resins, antioxidants, and various other ingredients. Surprisingly, chewing gum base has not been adequately tested for safety.

fd

CHLORINE
?

Chlorine is used by the baking industry for aging flour. Flour treated with chlorine seems to be safe for use in baked goods, however it has not been tested adequately.

fd

CHLORINE DIOXIDE
S

Chlorine dioxide is widely used by the baking industry as a bleaching and maturing agent. It proved to be a safe replacement for the chemical agene which was banned in 1949.

fd

CHLOROFORM
X

Measurable quantities of this poison can be found in our drinking water. Its presence is thought to be a result of chlorination of drinking water. Though the effects of the low levels of this toxic chemical in our water supplies are not known, it has been implicated in the two leading causes of death in the United States—cancer and cardiovascular disease.

env

CITRIC ACID, SODIUM CITRATE
S

Citric acid is one of the most widely used food additives. It is unquestionably safe. It is naturally present in virtually all living organisms and is found in high concentrations in berries and citrus fruits. It is used as an antioxidant to prevent spoiling in instant potatoes, canned fruits and vegetables, cheeses, candy, chewing gum, and many other products.

fd

CORN SYRUP
S

Corn syrup is a sweet, thick solution made from cornstarch. It is used as a sweetener and thickener mainly in low-nutrition foods. It is considered safe for human consumption, but it does promote tooth decay.

fd

CYSTEINE
S

Cysteine is a natural component of protein-containing foods. Small amounts are added to foods to prevent the breakdown of vitamin C.

fd

DEXTRIN
S

Dextrin is added to food products such as dried soup mixes as a thickening agent. This additive appears to be safe.

fd

DEXTROSE (GLUCOSE, CORN SUGAR)
S

This chemical is essential to all life as we know it. It is found in every cell of every living organism. Food manufacturers use dextrose mainly as a sweetener in a wide variety of foods. Though it is perfectly safe, high concentration of any sugar over a long period of time can lead to tooth decay. Don't overdo it.

fd

DIMETHYLPOLYSILOXANE (METHYL SILICONE, METHYL POLYSILICONE)
S

This substance is added to facilitate the manufacture of such foods as wine, refined sugar, yeast, and chewing gum. It has no harmful effects.

fd

DIOCTYL SODIUM SULFOSUCCINATE
S

This chemical is added to foods to facilitate the dissolving of powdered foods in water. It is widely used in powdered soft drink mixes and foods containing hard-to-dissolve thickening agents. It is safe at the levels found in foods.

fd

DISODIUM INOSINATE and DISODIUM GUANYLATE
S

These compounds are salts that have been derived from proteins. They are used as flavor enhancers. Research indicates that they are safe for human consumption.

fd

EDTA
?

EDTA is a chelating agent added to foods to trap trace amounts of metals that result from modern food-processing technology. These metal impurities would otherwise promote rancidity and the breakdown of artificial colors. It is found in salad dressings, margarine, sandwich spreads, processed fruits and vegetables, and soft drinks. Research has found it safe for human consumption in small quantities. However, when excess amounts accumulate in the body, EDTA can cause kidney damage and calcium imbalance.

fd

ERYTHORBIC ACID
S

Like vitamin C, erythorbic acid is added to foods to prevent loss of color and flavor. While it has no value as a nutrient, it is safe.

fd

FD&C BLUE 1
?

This is an artificial coloring found in many candies, baked goods, and beverages. Testing has been inadequate. It may be dangerous to health. Avoid it whenever possible.

fd

FD&C BLUE 2
?

This artificial coloring has not been proven to be safe. It should be avoided. It is found in beverages, candy, and pet food.

fd

FD&C GREEN 3
?

This coal-tar derivative is widely used as an artificial food coloring. It is recognized as safe by the Food and Drug Administration, yet has not been adequately tested. Avoid.

fd

FD&C ORANGE B
X

This artificial coloring is a good example of why consumers must be constantly on the alert. Orange B was approved by the FDA in 1966 as an artificial food coloring and was used in some hot dogs. In 1978 the producer stopped making it upon discovery that it contained a carcinogenic impurity.

fd

FD&C RED 3
?

This artificial food coloring is found is candy, baked goods, and in cherries in fruit cocktail. There is some suspicion that it may cause cancer. Since questions remain about its safety, it should be avoided.

fd

FD&C RED 4
X

High levels of this artificial coloring were found to cause damage to the adrenal cortex of dogs. After 1965 it was restricted to maraschino cherries and certain pills.

fd

FD&C RED 32
X

This artificial coloring was used in foods and drugs until 1956 when it was found to damage internal organs and was thought to be a weak cancer-causing agent. Since 1956 it has been used to color orange skins.

fd

FD&C RED 40
?

It is a widely used food coloring found in sausage, soft drinks, candy, and pastry. It has been associated with cancer in mice. It should be banned. Avoid it.

fd

FD&C YELLOW 5
?

This is the second most widely used food coloring. It is found in many products, including baked goods, candy, and pet foods. It has not been adequately tested. Until proved safe, it should be avoided.

fd

FD&C YELLOW 6
?

This artificial coloring is widely used in junk foods such as soft drinks and candy. It seems to be safe, but has been known to cause allergic reactions. It should probably be avoided.

fd

FERROUS GLUCONATE

S

This chemical is used by the olive industry to produce a uniformly colored black olive and is also used in some pills as a source of iron. It is safe for human consumption.

fd

FUMARIC ACID

S

This harmless food additive is an ideal source of tartness and acidity in dry food products such as powdered drinks, pumpkin-pie filling, and gelatin desserts. A variety of experiments have shown it to be harmless.

fd

FURCELLERAN

S

Furcelleran is a vegetable gum similar in properties to carrageen. It is a seaweed derivative used in many foods as a thickening and gelling agent. It is generally recognized as safe for human consumption.

fd

GELATIN

S

Gelatin is pure protein but has little nutritive value because it contains few or none of the essential amino acids. It is added to foods such as powdered dessert mixes, yogurt, and ice cream as a thickening and gelling agent. When gelatin is dissolved in hot water and allowed to cool, the protein molecules react with each other to form a gel. It is a safe additive.

fd

GLUCONIC ACID
S

Gluconic acid occurs naturally in the human body and is quite safe. It is occasionally used as a leavening agent in cake mixes.

fd

GLYCERIN (GLYCEROL)
S

This chemical is added to foods to maintain a certain moisture content and to prevent foods from drying out and becoming hard. Glycerin is used throughout the human body either as a source of energy or as a backbone for more complex molecules. It is perfectly safe. It is found in marshmallows, candy, fudge, and baked goods.

fd

GUMS
?

The class of food additives referred to as gums are derived from natural sources. They are generally used as thickening agents and stabilizers. Their safety has not been adequately tested. You should probably limit your intake of gums until their safety has been documented.

fd

GUM ARABIC (ACACIA GUM, GUM SENEGAL)
?

Food manufacturers use this vegetable gum to prevent

sugar crystals from forming in candy, to help citrus oils dissolve in drinks, to stabilize the foam in beer, and to improve the texture of ice cream. Its safety has not been adequately documented.

fd

GUM GHATTI
?

This vegetable gum is used by food processors to prevent oil and water ingredients from separating into two layers in such products as salad dressings. Its safety has not been tested.

fd

GUM GUAIAC
?

This greenish-brown resin is occasionally used by food processors to prevent oil-containing foods from spoiling. Its safety has not been adequately tested.

fd

GUAR GUM
?

Guar gum is one of the most widely used of the vegetable gum stabilizers. It is used as a thickening agent in beverages, ice cream, frozen pudding, and salad dressing. Guar gum has been shown to be digestible, but its safety has not been proved.

fd

HEPTYL PARABEN
?

This chemical is used as a preservative in some beers.

Though studies seem to indicate that it is a safe additive, it has not been fully tested—a good reason to cut down on your beer consumption.

fd

HYDROGENATED VEGETABLE OIL
?

Hydrogenated vegetable oil is used in margarine and many processed foods. When liquid vegetable oil is treated with hydrogen, it becomes a semisolid called hydrogenated vegetable oil. It converts polyunsaturated oils into saturated fats, which have been linked to heart disease. The typical American diet is already so high in saturated fats that hydrogenated vegetable oil should be avoided whenever possible.

fd

HYDROLYZED VEGETABLE PROTEIN (HVP)
S

HVP is added to foods to bring out their natural flavor. It is used in such products as instant soups, beef stews, frankfurters, gravy and sauce mixes, and canned chili. It is generally recognized as safe.

fd

HYDROXYLATED LECITHIN
?

Food manufacturers use hydroxylated lecithin as an emulsifier and an antioxidant or preservative in ice cream, baked goods, and margarine. The safety of this chemical additive has not been adequately documented. Until it is, its use should be limited.

fd

IMITATION BEEF and CHICKEN FLAVOR
?

Imitation beef and chicken flavors are made up of the following ingredients:

hydrolyzed vegetable protein
sugars
disodium inosate
disodium guanylate

monosodium glutamate
vegetable fats
amino acids
modified starch

See specific ingredients for safety rating.

fd

INVERT SUGAR
?

Invert sugar, a mixture of the sugars dextrose and fructose, is used as a sweetener in candy, soft drinks, and many other foods. Like all sugars, its use should be limited because it can lead to tooth decay.

fd

KARAYA GUM
?

Karaya gum is added to foods as a thickening or stabilizing agent. It is found in whipped products, salad dressings, ice cream, and sherbet. Because of its exceptional ability to absorb water, it is also used as a bulk laxative, a wave-set agent, and in various pharmaceuticals and cosmetics. Its safety has not been adequately documented.

fd

LACTIC ACID (CALCIUM LACTATE)
S

This chemical is found in all living things. It is added to

foods as an acidity regulator. It balances the acidity in cheese making and adds tartness to many foods such as carbonated drinks. It is safe.

fd

LACTOSE
S

Lactose is the sugar that is found naturally in milk. Food manufacturers use lactose, which is only one-sixth as sweet as table sugar, as a slightly sweet source of carbohydrate in breakfast pastry, whipped-topping mix, and many other foods. Lactose is a safe additive.

fd

LECITHIN
S

Lecithin is a nutritious, nontoxic, and important food additive. Lecithin is found in nearly all plant and animal tissues. Food manufacturers add lecithin to margarines, shortenings, and oils to retard spoilage. It is also added to chocolate, ice cream, and baked goods to promote the mixing of oil and water. The safety of lecithin has been proven.

fd

LOCUST BEAN GUM (CAROB SEED GUM, ST. JOHN'S BREAD)
?

This derivative of the bean of the carob tree is added to food as a stabilizer. It is used to improve the texture of ice cream, to thicken salad dressings and barbecue sauces, and as a dough additive to produce thicker and softer cakes and biscuits. The safety of locust bean gum has not been adequately tested.

fd

MALIC ACID
S

Malic acid is present in all living cells. It has been widely used by the food manufacturing industry as a flavoring agent in fruit-flavored drinks, candy, lemon-flavored ice tea mix, and ice cream. It is safe.

fd

MALTOL, ETHYL MALTOL
?

These additives, used to bring out the flavor of fruit-, vanilla-, and chocolate-flavored foods, are assumed to be free of agents that cause cancer, birth defects, or mutations, but they have not been proven completely safe. They should be avoided until they are adequately tested.

fd

MANNITOL
S

This substance which occurs naturally in the manna ash tree is useful to food manufacturers because it doesn't absorb water, is sweet, and is poorly absorbed by the body. Mannitol is used as the "dust" on chewing gum to prevent the gum from absorbing moisture. Since only 50 percent of it can be absorbed by the body, mannitol is used as a sweetener in low-calorie foods and in sugarless gum. Mannitol has been safely used by humans for centuries.

fd

MELENGESTROL ACETATE (MGA)
?

This is a female hormone injected into some cattle to reduce their sex drive, to prevent the loss of valuable pounds caused by engaging in sexual activity. Trace amounts of this female hormone can be found in some of the meat that reaches your table. It effect on health has not been tested.

fd

MONO- and DIGLYCERIDES
S

These chemical additives are used to make baked goods softer, improve the stability of margarine, and prevent the separation of oil from peanut butter. The average American probably consumes a half-pound of these chemicals each year as food additives. Mono- and diglycerides have been found harmless.

fd

MONOSODIUM GLUTAMATE
?

Monosodium glutamate (MSG) is used throughout the world by consumers and food manufacturers to bring out the flavor of protein-containing foods. It is the active ingredient in the oriental condiments soy sauce and sea tangle. MSG has been known to cause "Chinese restaurant syndrome" (burning sensation in the back of the neck and forearms, tightness of the chest, and headaches). Though doctors believe that Chinese restaurant syndrome is only a minor annoyance with no lasting effects, ingestion of large amounts of MSG has been found to result in destruction of nerve cells in the brains of newborn laboratory animals.

Thus pregnant women should limit their intake of MSG.

fd

PARABENS
S

Parabens are chemicals that are added to foods and pharmaceutical products as preservatives. Parabens appear to be safe.

fd

PECTIN
S

Pectin is a natural component of many foods such as fruits and vegetables. It is added to foods to thicken gels, barbecue sauce, cranberry sauce, canned frosting, and yogurt. It is perfectly safe.

fd

PHOSPHORIC ACID, PHOSPHATES
?

These are found in such products as baked goods, soft drinks, cheese, powdered foods, cured meat, breakfast cereals, and dehydrated potatoes. They are used to acidify cola beverages; as mineral supplements, buffers, and emulsifiers; and to inhibit discoloration. They are safe as food additives, but are so widely used that they may lead to a nutritional imbalance that causes osteoporosis, soft or brittle bones. Limit your intake of phosphoric acid and phosphates.

fd

PHOSPHOROUS
?

Phosphorous is used in the processing of poultry, in the production of soft drinks, and in the production of modified starches. An excessive daily intake of phosphorous can lead to premature slowing of bone growth in children.

env

POLYSORBATE 60
S

This is an emulsifier added to such foods as baked goods, frozen desserts, and imitation dairy products. It keeps baked goods from going stale, helps nondairy creamers dissolve in coffee, and prevents oils from separating out of frozen desserts. It appears to be safe at the levels normally consumed in foods.

fd

POTASSIUM CARBONATE, SODIUM CARBONATE
S

These additives are used in such products as dried soup mixes to neutralize acidity. They have been found safe.

fd

PROPYL GALLATE
X

Propyl gallate is an antioxidant or preservative, often used in combination with BHA and BHT because they work together to retain freshness. It has not been adequately tested for safety and therefore should be avoided. There are safer antioxidants that should be used in its place.

fd

PROPYLENE GLYCOL
S

This food additive is an emulsifier used in such products as soup mixes to help maintain desired texture. It represents no hazard.

fd

SACCHARIN
X

Saccharin is an artificial sweetener three- to five-hundred times sweeter than sugar. Because the body does not convert saccharin to glucose, it is used by persons suffering from diabetes as an alternative to sugar. It is also the main sweetener used in low-calorie foods and drinks. There is some evidence that saccharin may cause cancer. Be safe—read and follow the warning label printed on artificially sweetened products: "Saccharin is a sweetener which should be used only by persons who must restrict their intake of ordinary sweets."

fd

SALICYLATES
X

Used in synthetic flavorings and dyes and in analgesic tablets, they may cause hyperkinesis in children. Fifteen percent of reported deaths in children under six are due to salicylates in analgesic tablets. They may cause degenerative change in kidneys, brain, lungs, and liver.

fd

SILICON DIOXIDE
S

Silicon dioxide is a stabilizer, anticaking agent, and thickener. It is safe.

fd

SODIUM BENZOATE
S

Sodium benzoate is used as a preservative in acidic foods such as fruit juices, carbonated drinks, pickles, salad dressings, and preserves. All evidence indicates that it is safe.

fd

SODIUM BISULFITE, SULFUR DIOXIDE
?

Sodium bisulfite and sulfur dioxide gas are added to foods to prevent discoloration and to inhibit the growth of bacteria. They are used in carbonated drinks, wine, grape juice, sliced fruits, and vegetables, among other foods. Bisulfite destroys vitamin B-1, therefore continued consumption of foods treated with this chemical could lead to a vitamin deficiency. Otherwise, they are safe.

fd

SODIUM CARBOXYMETHYLCELLULOSE (CMC)
S

CMC is used as a thickening and stabilizing agent in ice cream, beer, pie fillings, diet foods, and candy. It is safe.

fd

SODIUM ERYTHROBATE
?

Sodium erythrobate is added to processed meats to retard color fading and improve appearance. It is found in frankfurters, bologna, pastrami, and other cured meats. Studies testing its safety as a food additive have been inadequate. Avoid it.

fd

SODIUM NITRITE, SODIUM NITRATE

X

Nitrite is one of the few food additives that is definitely known to have caused deaths in the United States. It is toxic at levels only moderately higher than those found in foods on your supermarket shelf. Nitrites and nitrates are also dangerous because they can be converted into cancer-causing chemicals called nitrosamines during cooking and in the body. They are added to foods such as bacon, ham, frankfurters, and luncheon meats to prevent the growth of bacteria that causes botulism. Avoid these foods.

fd

SODIUM SILICO ALUMINATE

S

This is an alkaline anticaking agent. It is used in dried products such as soup mixes to keep the mix free-flowing. Research has found it safe.

fd

SOFT WATER

?

Research has found that people who live in an area supplied with soft drinking water are significantly more likely to suffer from heart disease. Scientists are currently trying to determine the reasons.

env

SORBIC ACID, POTASSIUM SORBATE

S

Sorbic acid, which occurs naturally in the berries of the mountain ash, is used to prevent the growth of mold and bacteria in such foods as cheese, syrup, jelly, baked goods, wine, and dry fruits. It appears to be safe.

fd

SORBITAN MONOSTEARATE
S

This food additive is used in baked goods, candy, frozen pudding, and icing as an emulsifier to keep oil and water mixed together. Research indicates that it is safe.

fd

SORBITOL
S

Sorbitol is added to products such as candy, shredded coconut, chewing gum, and dietetic foods and drinks as a sweetener and thickening agent. Research has shown it to be safe in the small amounts used in foods. It is also safe for use by diabetics because it is absorbed slowly and does not cause blood sugar to rise rapidly.

fd

STARCH, MODIFIED STARCH
?

Starch, the major component of many foods such as potatoes and corn, and its chemical counterpart, modified starch, are used to make foods such as soups and gravies look thicker and richer than they really are. Starch is normally thought of as a food and is a wholesome and safe additive. We do not, however, feel that the safety of modified starch has been proven and recommend that you limit your intake of this additive.

fd

TANNIN
?

Tannin is found in coffee, tea, and cocoa. Food manufacturers add tannin to butter, caramel, fruit, brandy, maple, and nut artificial flavorings. Tannin is suspected of being a weak cancer-causing chemical. Avoid it or limit your intake.

fd

TARTARIC ACID
S

Tartaric acid is found naturally in grapes and other fruits. It is added to beverages, candy, ice cream, baked goods, and other foods because of its tart taste. It is safe.

fd

TEXTURED VEGETABLE PROTEIN (TVP)
?

Textured vegetable protein is soy protein that has been treated with chemical additives and processed into portions that resemble meat. Since the nutritional value of soy protein is similar to that of meat protein, products made with TVP are unquestionably nutritious. The problem with TVP lies in the nature of the chemical additives it is combined with. Before you use any product made with TVP read the label and make sure the additives used with it are safe.

fd

THIODIPROPIONIC ACID, DILAURYL THIODIPROPIONATE

?

These chemicals are sometimes used in food and food packaging to prevent fats and oils from spoiling. Studies designed to test their safety have not been adequate. Avoid.

fd

VANILLIN, ETHYL VANILLIN

S, ?

Vanillin and ethyl vanillin are cheaper synthetic substitutes for the flavoring, vanilla. They are used in ice cream, baked goods, beverages, chocolate, and candy among other products. Vanillin has been found to be harmless; ethyl vanillin has not been adequately tested for safety.

fd

INDEX